the
CLEVER GUT DIET
cookbook

Disclaimer: This publication contains the opinions and ideas of its author. It is intended to provide helpful and informative material on the subjects addressed in the publication. It is not intended as and should not be relied upon as medical advice. It is sold with the understanding that the author and publisher are not engaged in rendering medical, health, or any other kind of personal professional services in the book. The reader should consult his or her medical, health, or other competent professional before adopting any of the suggestions in this book or drawing inferences from it. The author and publisher specifically disclaim all responsibility for any liability, loss or risk, personal or otherwise, which is incurred as a consequence, directly or indirectly, of the use and application of any of the contents of this book.

ATRIA
PAPERBACK

An Imprint of Simon & Schuster, Inc.
1230 Avenue of the Americas
New York, NY 10020

Copyright © 2017 by Parenting Matters Ltd
Photographs copyright © 2017 by Joe Sarah
Originally published in Great Britain in 2017 by Short Books
Published by arrangement with Short Books Limited

All rights reserved, including the right to reproduce this book or portions thereof in any form whatsoever. For information, address Atria Books Subsidiary Rights Department, 1230 Avenue of the Americas, New York, NY 10020.

First Atria Paperback edition May 2018

ATRIA PAPERBACK and colophon are trademarks of Simon & Schuster, Inc.

For information about special discounts for bulk purchases, please contact Simon & Schuster Special Sales at 1-866-506-1949 or business@simonandschuster.com.

The Simon & Schuster Speakers Bureau can bring authors to your live event. For more information or to book an event, contact the Simon & Schuster Speakers Bureau at 1-866-248-3049 or visit our website at www.simonspeakers.com.

Manufactured in the United States of America

10   9   8   7   6   5   4   3   2   1

Library of Congress Cataloging-in-Publication Data
Names: Bailey, Clare, author.
Title: The clever gut diet recipe book : delicious recipes to help you nourish your body from the inside out / Dr. Clare Bailey with nutritionist Joy Skipper.
Description: First Atria Paperback edition. | New York, NY : Atria Paperback, 2018. | Originally published in Great Britain in 2017 by Short Books. | Includes bibliographical references and index.
Identifiers: LCCN 2017052701 (print) | LCCN 2017053947 (ebook)
Subjects: LCSH: Weight loss. | Reducing diets—Recipes. | Digestive Organs—Diseases—Diet therapy. | BISAC: COOKING / Health & Healing / Weight Control. | HEALTH & FITNESS / Diets. | HEALTH & FITNESS / Weight Loss.
Classification: LCC RM222.2 (ebook) | LCC RM222.2 .B3424 2018 (print) | DDC 641.5/63—dc23
LC record available at https://lccn.loc.gov/2017052701

ISBN 978-1-5011-8976-0
ISBN 978-1-5011-8977-7 (ebook)

the CLEVER GUT DIET cookbook

150 delicious recipes to help you
nourish your body from the inside out

Dr. Clare Bailey WITH
nutritionist Joy Skipper

FOREWORD BY DR. MICHAEL MOSLEY

ATRIA PAPERBACK
New York London Toronto Sydney New Delhi

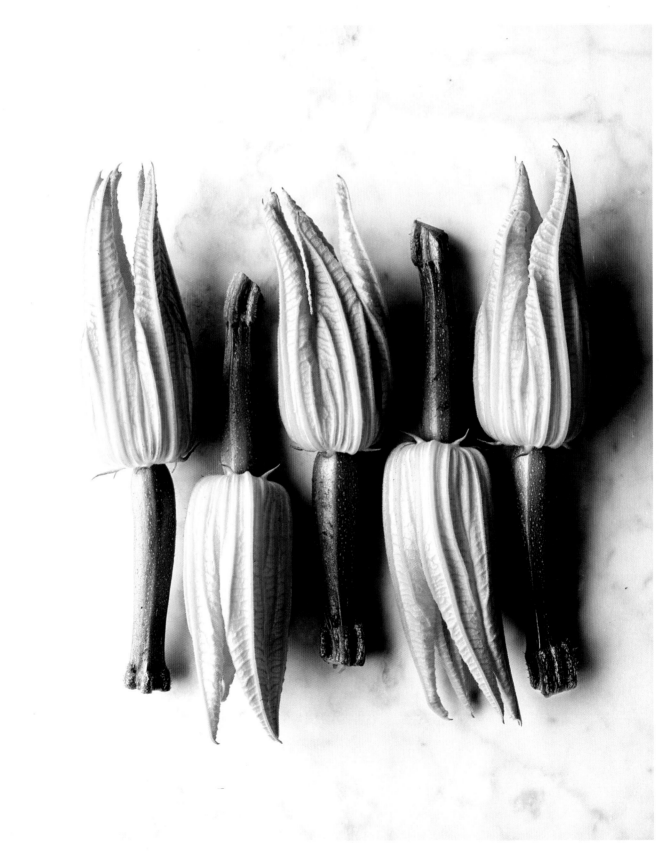

Contents

Foreword by Dr. Michael Mosley 6

Introduction by Dr. Clare Bailey 8

The Clever Gut Diet 10

1 Breakfast 30

2 Light Meals, Soups, and Salads 52

3 Dressings and Flavorings 114

4 Main Dishes 124

5 Clever Vegetables 158

6 Ferments 178

7 Treats 192

Meal Planners 214

Acknowledgments 218

Index 219

Foreword by Dr. Michael Mosley

Hippocrates, the father of modern medicine, claimed over 2,000 years ago that "all diseases begin in the gut." It's taken a long time, but we are beginning to realize just how profound Hippocrates' insight really was. There's never been as much interest in the human gut and its tiny inhabitants, the trillions of microbes that make up the microbiome, as there is now. New research tools have enabled scientists to probe the previously secret world of the gut, and uncover more and more about the impact that the 1,000 different species that live down there have on you, and you have on them. Thanks to advances in DNA technology, we have learned more surprising things about the gut in the last few years than in all of previous human history. It's been a bit like Galileo inventing the telescope and using it to discover a whole new universe, one that is larger and more complex than anything that earlier generations could ever have imagined.

These new discoveries about the gut are not just of academic interest. It is becoming ever clearer just how important the microbiome is for keeping the rest of our body, and brain, in good shape. We have recently learned, for example, that the mix of microbes in our gut can strongly influence our weight, our mood, and even our immune system. The tragedy is that a modern diet, which relies heavily on processed food, along with the widespread overuse of antibiotics, has laid waste to the modern microbiome. This helps explain some of the dramatic increases we've seen over the last few decades in obesity, type 2 diabetes, allergic diseases, and food intolerances.

What's the link? Well, an addiction to junk food and the indiscriminate use of antibiotics have helped devastate our "Old Friends." These are the microbes that live in our guts and which evolved with us. They are essential to our health. Devastating these Old Friends has in turn made space for unhealthy microbes to flourish, those that encourage inflammation, weight gain, and, possibly, depression.

The good news is that it's never too late to do something to help those Old Friends recover. Adding new foods to your diet, doing a bit more exercise, and simply getting outdoors more can all have a positive impact on your gut health.

This book is only possible because of the extraordinary work done by scientists from many different countries who have generously shared their time and research. But it is also a labor of love by its main author, Dr. Clare Bailey. I have known Clare for over 35 years. We met on our first day of medical school and married soon after graduating. As well as being a dedicated doctor, Clare has always been passionate and adventurous about food. When she was working with the Save the Children Fund in a remote part of the Amazon jungle, she was fascinated as much by her medical work there as by the unusual foods they were eating. This included, on one occasion, a giant toad, "as large as a chicken," which they shared between four people. Apparently it was delicious.

These days Clare is a busy GP who, among other things, uses her love of food and interest in nutrition to help her patients improve their blood sugar levels and reverse their type 2 diabetes by losing weight, rather than relying on medication. This led to her writing the bestselling *8-Week Blood Sugar Diet Cookbook*.

Building on what she has learned, she is now using food to improve her patients' gut health as well as their gut size. The recipes in this book are the product of the latest science. They are gut-friendly, but taste, flavor, and simplicity are equally important. They are also written with a busy person in mind, so the ingredients should be easy to access and inexpensive.

I have greatly enjoyed eating my way through the recipes in this book and I hope you do, too.

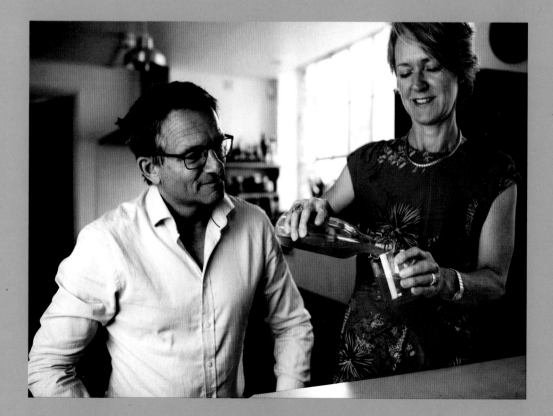

Introduction by Dr. Clare Bailey

I have been working as a doctor for over 30 years and in that time have seen a lot of remarkable medical changes and innovations. But to discover a whole new world, a new organ, if you like, one that produces chemicals, controls our appetites, moods, and metabolism, that can work for us or against us depending on how we treat it . . . this really is a new frontier. We are starting to discover this new world's many inhabitants, and to learn what they do, what disturbs them, and how they can be nurtured or defeated. Welcome to the microbiome, the trillions of microbes that live in your intestines.

This book will introduce you to some of these tiny guys busily working away to keep you happy and healthy. More importantly, it will show you how you can help them help you, how you can feed them the variety of fiber and nutrients they need and increase their numbers with probiotics, the healthy microbes found in fermented foods.

In recent decades, we have abandoned traditional ways of eating, relying on instant and processed foods, which more often than not are high in sugars. In the UK the average adult eats some 200 sandwiches a year, and the most common choice of filling is cheese, followed closely by ham. A limited diet of this nature is bound to have a negative impact on our health and particularly on our gut health. Nor is it enough to live on a "healthy" diet of avocados, sweet potatoes, bagged spinach, and cherry tomatoes and think you've got it sorted out . . .

Like us, our microbiome thrives on variety, which is why the recipes here offer a diverse range of proteins, whether plant-based, seafood, or meat. It is why we encourage you to eat vegetables of every color and try new foods and flavors.

You may be reading this book because you have trouble with your gut. Perhaps you suspect a food intolerance or that you have Irritable Bowel Syndrome (IBS), and feel that your gut is in need of a reboot (see page 24). Or maybe you are doing this simply to broaden your horizons and improve your diet with some gut-friendly recipes—in which case try as many as you can. This is not a diet focused on weight loss, though this can happen as part of the process, particularly if you incorporate the 5:2 approach (see page 18).

As someone who loves experimenting with food, I hope most of all that you enjoy the meals we have put together and that they make you feel well and content with life.

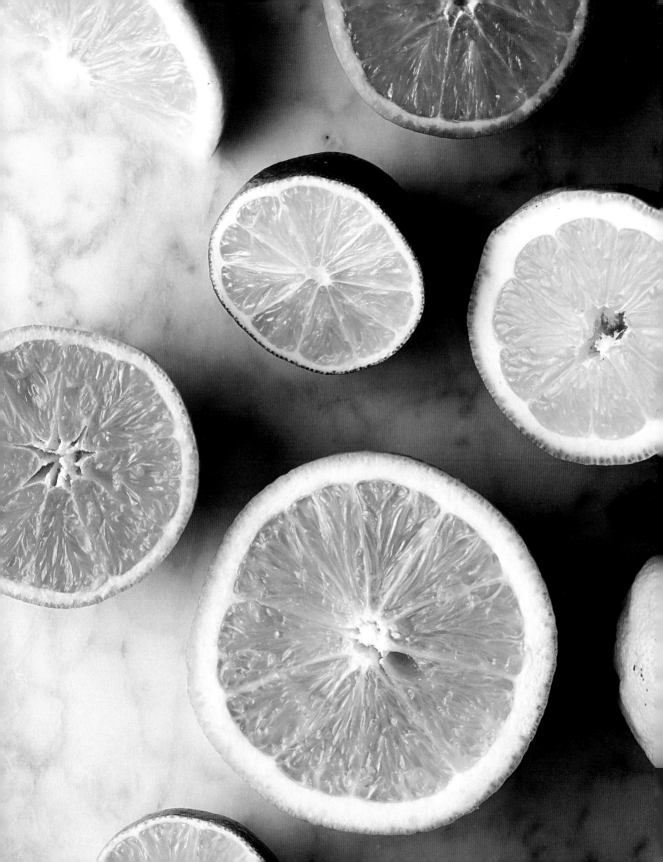

The Clever Gut Diet

Based on the Mediterranean way of eating

This diet is based on "real food"—plenty of vegetables, fruits, nuts, beans, olive oil, cheese, meat, and fatty fish, but relatively little starchy pizza, pasta, potatoes, or bread. We call it "Mediterranean style" because although many of the recipes have a Mediterranean twist, they draw on healthy cuisines from all over the world. Most of the ingredients you will be familiar with; some (such as fermented foods and seaweed) will be more surprising. Where it is convenient we go back to more traditional ways of preparation that may have been lost in the era of fast, processed, and packaged foods. That said, none of the recipes are particularly complicated or time-consuming. The emphasis is on freshness, good flavors, and being "doable." I have plenty of patients who don't particularly like to cook and I keep them in mind when I am creating recipes. We recommend using natural single ingredients where possible: That way you know what is in your food and don't have to decipher the secret code words of a dozen or more added ingredients.

We love this diet because as well as being incredibly tasty, it is the best researched on the planet. Big studies have shown that compared to a diet that is low in fat and high in starchy carbs, this form of Mediterranean diet—based on eating fairly low Glycemic Index (GI) foods which tend to be higher in fiber and release sugars more slowly—will help you keep the weight off, halve your risk of developing type 2 diabetes, reduce your risk of developing cancer (particularly breast cancer), and keep your brain in good shape. Last but by no means least, it will help you maintain a healthy microbiome.

Low in sugars and starchy carbohydrates

Eating lots of white carbs and sugary, processed foods will not only damage your waistline, but your microbiome as well. These foods will encourage the growth of unhealthy microbes, which in turn cause inflammation.

The problem is that sugars and starchy carbs are everywhere, not just in the obvious items like soda, cookies, and donuts. They are in pretty much every processed food you buy—often listed as separate ingredients, such as glucose, maltose syrup, maltodextrin, dextrose, fruit juice concentrates, corn fructose, high fructose corn syrup, malt syrup, raw sugar, lactose, cane sugar . . . There are over 60 different names that may appear on food labels, most of them sounding fairly innocuous. Another reason to avoid processed foods if you can.

Retrain your palate and your microbiome by cutting back on sugar. Believe it or not, as your gut biome changes, the cravings will fade. Feeding the good microbes with a healthy diet will gradually silence the messages being sent out by the sugar-loving ones that are calling for more. You should notice a difference within a few weeks.

Skip the artificial sweeteners, too—these cheat your system into expecting a sugar fix and help maintain your sweet tooth (they're often many times sweeter-tasting than the real stuff). They can also damage a healthy microbiome. Kick the habit and your tastes will change. You will become more sensitive to other flavors and enjoy much lower levels of sugar, or even start finding it cloying and slightly sickly. (See chapter 7 for low-sugar treats.)

Choose more vegetables—try and ensure they take up at least half a plate. Make them interesting and varied. Add butter or olive oil. Pep them up with flavorings such as red pepper flakes, cumin, or a squeeze of lemon. Stir-fry your greens. Add garlic. If you are not a great fan of vegetables, start your meal with them, so that you are eating them when you are hungry. They may become your favorite part of the meal. Michael used to shuffle his vegetables around his plate with little interest. He now even adds extra—and consumes far fewer starchy carbs as a result. (See chapter 5 for vegetable dishes.)

Get your digestive juices going with a light, enzyme-inducing salad at the beginning of your meal to improve your digestion (see page 55).

Focused on good food not calories

We have included calories as an aid, not as a focus. The main reason they are recorded is to help those who are including a 5:2 intermittent fasting element in their diet (see page 18) as this has been shown to improve gut health as well as increase weight loss and boost the metabolism. The calories are recorded per portion unless otherwise stated. They are also rounded to the nearest zero. Don't get too caught up on them. Whatever the calorie content of the food you put in your mouth, the mix of microbes in your gut will help decide what proportion of it is absorbed. Some people have much more calorie-rich stool than others. Different foods behave differently, depending on how you prepare them and what you eat them with. So, for example, eating a baked potato is likely to raise your blood sugar less if you add butter or cheese. Who would have guessed?

Food Groups and the Microbiome

Protein

As protein cannot be stored, the average adult needs to eat 45-60g of it a day. However, unless you are doing very physical work or extreme amounts of exercise, more is not necessarily better. This is a moderate-protein diet, not a high-protein diet.

Variety is all when it comes to gut health, so eat as broad a range of protein as you can. Quality proteins include meat, fatty fish, eggs, seafood, tofu, and cheese. Other good sources include edamame, Quorn, nuts, and tempeh. There are strong ethical reasons why you might want to avoid meat, but it is undoubtedly an excellent source of protein and important nutrients such as iron. We recommend eating free-range meat if possible. Eat less, but better quality—ideally red meat no more than twice a week. It is advised to restrict processed meats (such as salami and bacon) as they are more likely to contain additives, preservatives, or hydrogenated oils.

Healthy natural fats

These are found in plant foods, such as nuts, seeds, olive oil, and avocados, and in dairy products, as well as meat and seafood—fatty fish being one of the best sources. Increasing the proportion of healthy fats you eat helps to reset your metabolism and reduce blood sugar. Fat slows the release of starchy carbohydrates and sugars (hence the baked potato conundrum at the end of the last section). Being slow to burn, it provides a steady source of energy that doesn't stimulate the release of insulin (the fat storage hormone). That said, there are fats that you should try to avoid—the trans and partially hydrogenated fats that are mainly present in spreads and processed foods, such as cookies and pastries.

Dairy

Foods such as yogurt and cheese are an excellent source of calcium and protein, and are not the demons responsible for increasing the risk of developing heart disease or type 2 diabetes that we once thought they were. However, dairy products contain the sugar lactose, which can cause digestive symptoms, such as bloating, cramps, and diarrhea. Around 75 percent of the world's population are lactose-intolerant, and if you have it mildly you may not have identified it as the cause of your symptoms. If this is the case, it may be worth trying a brief exclusion diet to see if it helps (as described in Phase 1—see page 25). We do include dairy products in many of the recipes, but suggest alternatives, such as nut or soy products, wherever possible.

Grains

We are not anti-grain by any means; in fact, whole grains are found to be beneficial. But because many grains contain gluten, which can irritate the gut and in some people cause problems, we have tried to minimize using it in our recipes. We have used traditional, lower-gluten grains, such as rye or spelt, and "artisan" bread-making techniques such as sourdough, where the fermentation process breaks down much of the gluten, making it easier to tolerate.

For those who are avoiding gluten altogether, many gluten-free flours are now available. They are made with a blend of ingredients, such as rice flour, potato flour, and tapioca, and are designed for baking. However, they are often white and highly refined, and tend to lack the healthy fiber needed by your microbiome. We would urge you where possible to use whole grain alternatives such as buckwheat flour, which, despite the misleading name, is gluten-free, or whole grain chickpea flour, also known as gram flour or besan, or indeed nut flours or ground almonds, which are also high in protein and healthy natural oils. There are lots of tricks to help produce a bread-like texture or softer cakes, such as adding xanthan gum.

Fiber

Fiber acts like a broom for the digestive system, helping the gut to push waste through the intestine. It is broadly made up of non-digestible carbohydrates and acts as a source of energy and nutrients for the creatures that live in your gut. We should all be aiming to eat at least 35g of fiber a day; unfortunately, the average Western diet contains less than half of that.

Most foods contain a mix of soluble and insoluble fiber. Soluble fiber attracts water and partially dissolves, forming a thick gel which helps to create the stool and move it through the intestines. It can also help reduce heart disease. Soluble fiber is found in foods like oatmeal, barley, lentils, beans, potatoes, carrots, bananas, avocados, and okra.

Insoluble fiber doesn't dissolve; it is more "scratchy" and adds bulk to the stool. Two of the most important types of it, as far as your gut is concerned, are inulin and fructooligosaccharides. These are prebiotics, which are not digested in the small intestine, but continue on down the gut to become an important source of nutrients for the microbiome, promoting the growth of beneficial bacteria. These bacteria, through fermentation of fiber in the colon, produce the vital short-chain fatty acids, such as butyrate, propionate and acetate, which in turn play an important role in health and disease. Fructooligosaccharides are also a natural sweetener.

Insoluble fiber is found in foods such as asparagus, chicory, Jerusalem artichokes, onions, string beans, wheat bran, celery, and tough stems of cabbage or kale. In some people it can exacerbate symptoms of IBS, so we include less of this in Phase 1 recipes.

Prebiotics and probiotics

Prebiotics are non-digestible carbohydrates, usually fiber, that have beneficial effects, particularly through encouraging the growth of gut-friendly micro-organisms. They are like the fertilizer that helps the grass grow in a lawn.

Probiotics are like the seeds that you scatter on the lawn to keep it lush and compete with the weeds. They are "friendly" live bacteria, found naturally in fermented foods such as sauerkraut, kefir, and yogurt (see chapter 6), which work in a variety of ways along the digestive tract, boosting healthy microbes and driving down numbers of the harmful ones. We love them!

Polyphenols and phytonutrients

Polyphenols are the most common antioxidants in our food and tend to be found in plant fiber. They have anti-inflammatory properties and are good for your gut health as well as for your brain and heart. As much as 90-95% of the polyphenol-rich foods you take in make it down to the colon, where they are processed by microbes and encourage the growth of beneficial bacteria. Herbs, spices, nuts, seeds, berries, teas, red wine, and dark chocolate contain high quantities of polyphenols, and we have included many of these in our recipes.

Phytonutrients are natural components of plants that keep them healthy, protecting them from disease and damage. Their antioxidant and anti-inflammatory properties also provide significant health benefits and help to preserve a healthy microbial balance in the gut. Phytonutrients are concentrated in the pigments in the skin of fruit and vegetables, so the key is to eat a wide variety of colors—aim for two or more of each per day.

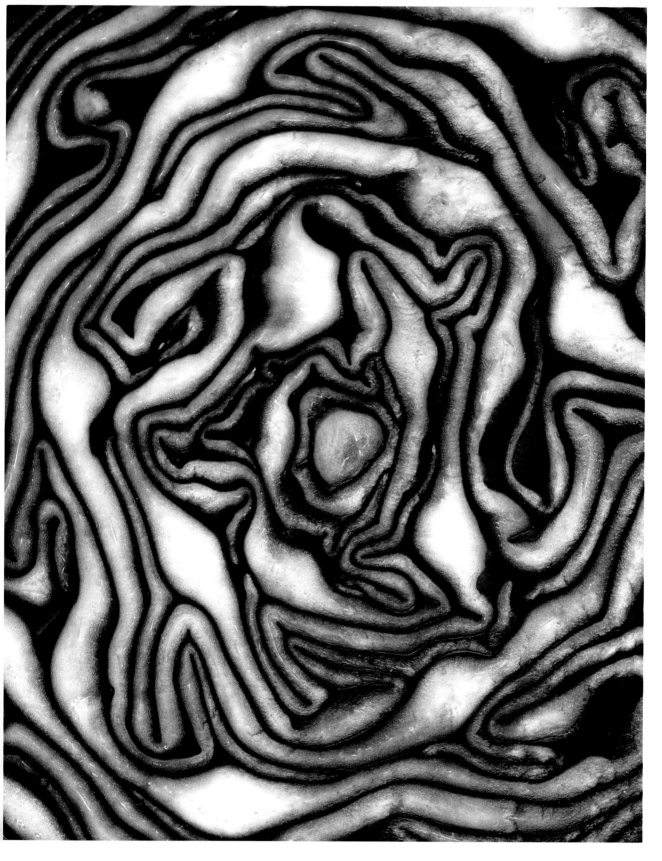

Ten Gut-Friendly
Foods and Why
We Love Them

1. Olive oil. As well as adding flavor and taste—and being safe to cook with—olive oil is one of the healthiest fats you can eat, rich in a range of polyphenols and antioxidants which are good at damping down inflammation.

2. Fatty fish. Like olive oil, fatty fish is full of good fats. The key ingredient is omega-3s. Unfortunately, white fish, like cod, don't contain many omega-3 fatty acids and don't provide the same health benefits.

3. Nuts. Nuts have had a bad rap because they are fatty and high in calories. However, there is very good evidence that the odd handful of nuts, eaten as a snack, will cut your risk of heart disease. They are also high in protein and fiber, and satiating.

4. Full-fat active Greek-style yogurt. Not only tasty and filling, this form of yogurt is also rich in health-inducing bacteria like *Lactobacillus*. The evidence that full-fat is better for you than low-fat is compelling. Plenty of studies have found that regularly eating full-fat yogurt leads to less weight gain and a lower risk of diseases such as type 2 diabetes.

5. Vegetables and fruit. Everyone knows that fruits and vegetables are good for us, but even those who eat their five a day tend to stick to a very limited range. And that means our microbiome ends up being pretty limited as well. A simple solution is to add more color to your plate . . .

6. Eggs. Not so long ago we were warned not to eat more than a couple of eggs a week, yet it turns out that the fear of cholesterol in eggs was totally misplaced. Eggs are a superb source of protein and rich in vitamins and minerals.

7. Fermented foods. Fermentation occurs when microbes in the food convert sugars into other compounds. The unique flavors and textures in them are due to the different species of bacteria and yeasts. Wine, cheese, yogurt, and chocolate are all fermented foods, as are kimchi, sauerkraut, kefir, kombucha, pickles, and miso. The microbes in fermented foods are also far more likely than most other bacteria to make it safely down into your colon because they are extremely resistant to acid, having been reared in an acidic environment.

8. Turmeric. Turmeric contains at least 200 different compounds, but the one that's of particular interest to scientists is called curcumin. Evidence shows that turmeric has powerful antioxidant and anti-inflammatory properties, is good at inhibiting the growth of "bad" bacteria and fungi, and indirectly protects the wall of the intestine.

9. Raw unfiltered apple cider vinegar. This is another fermented food that is now hugely popular. A shot of apple cider vinegar taken before breakfast reduces blood sugar levels and there is evidence that it can also reduce cholesterol.

10. Seaweed. Seaweed is rich in fiber, packed with nutrients, and has been shown to lead to a significant reduction in inflammation and an increase in insulin sensitivity.

Intermittent Fasting and Gut Health

We now know that intermittent fasting—short periods of reducing your calorie intake—improves your metabolic markers beyond those expected for weight loss. It also reduces blood sugar levels, leads to improvements in the lining of the gut, and boosts the health of the microbiome. Giving your gut a rest from having to constantly digest food allows the lining to regenerate and encourages the growth of good bacteria like *Akkermansia*.

There are various ways of practicing intermittent fasting—from simply increasing your overnight fast to 12-14 hours, to doing prolonged periods of 800-calorie fasting as Michael outlines in *The 8-Week Blood Sugar Diet*, or the popular 5:2 fasting approach that he sets out in *The FastDiet* (5 days eating normally, 2 days on 500-600 calories).

We have included many recipes for those of you who are intermittent fasting—with an updated regimen of 800-calorie fast days. If you like the look of the higher-calorie recipes but want to lose weight, we would recommend on fast days having half the stated portion and adding more vegetables.

Simply avoiding snacks is the minimum "fasting" you could do. Most snacks prevent your body from going into fat-burning mode and cheat your microbiome of the chance to repair the gut lining between meals. If you must snack, choose unsalted, unflavored nuts. Or snack on chopped vegetables or even a small amount of dark chocolate (at least 70% cocoa solids).

Tips for your 800-calorie 5:2 fasting days

- **Plan fasting days** in advance.

- **Make sure you increase your water intake** as you miss out on the fluids in your usual food and you lose water when you burn fat. Aim for 8-12 cups a day.

- **Soups are surprisingly satiating, cheap, and practical.** They are also more slowly digested. You can take them to work for lunch and keep portions in the freezer. Go for the non-starchy vegetable or clear broths like Quick Seaweed Miso Soup (page 61).

- **Drinking hot drinks suppresses appetite:** teas, coffee, or Turmeric Tea (see page 21).

- **Use flavor enhancers** so each meal is as tasty as possible, for example lemon, pepper, lime, chiles, garlic, pickles, mustard, herbs. They add very little in terms of calories.

- **Monitor blood sugar regularly if you are diabetic:** ideally twice daily at different times of the day at first. Consult your doctor before you begin the diet.

- **Side effects:** tiredness, lightheadedness, and headaches (these are often related to dehydration), hunger (this comes in waves and passes so try to "surf the wave"), and feeling colder. All of these should settle over a week or so and are usually less noticeable if you increase the amount of fat you eat in your diet.

- **Avoid fasting or discuss with your doctor first if:** your BMI is below 20, you have a history of eating disorders, are under 18 years of age, are on medication, are pregnant or breastfeeding, have a significant psychiatric disorder, are ill or have a significant medical condition, are recovering from surgery, are frail, or have other medical conditions.

The first few weeks can be tough, but your body adapts. Your appetite settles. In fact most people feel better and find they have more energy and a clearer head. It helps to get support. The website thebloodsugardiet.com provides plenty of useful resources and the opportunity to join a supportive, well-informed community.

Establishing Healthy Habits

Try to use this book to build healthy habits, whether you are hoping to improve your gut health and digestion or simply want to feel your best. One of the most important things you can do, right at the start, is involve other people. Tell your friends and family what you're planning and what you hope to achieve. Try to persuade one of them to join you, because being part of something bigger means you are more likely to succeed. Join an online community (such as cleverguts.com) for advice and support.

If, despite your best intentions, you find you are struggling, question your excuses. What is getting in the way? It can be uncomfortable making changes but stick with it and your better habits will become automatic.

Plan ahead—this helps to bypass "willpower," which is usually in short supply and easily gets used up. Practice a bit of kitchen hygiene—remove temptations from your surfaces and cupboards. Research has shown that people who live in households with cereal boxes or cookies on view are more likely to be overweight than those who keep them in the cupboards, out of sight.

If you are watching your weight, practice portion control. Use a smaller plate, eat slowly, and listen to your appetite. This will give your body time to send the message that you are full. If you have raised blood sugar, these vital feedback loops stop working, leaving you constantly hungry and unsatisfied. It's not greed, just the system out of kilter. If you stick with it, your blood sugar levels should improve and the normal feedback system will reestablish itself, leaving you feeling comfortably full after eating. My patients often say that after the first week or two it gets much easier.

Get up a bit earlier—10 more minutes gives you time to make a healthy swap from toast and jam or processed cereals to a delicious and filling breakfast, such as scrambled eggs or oatmeal (see chapter 1 for more breakfast suggestions).

Get to bed earlier—better sleep enhances concentration, resets your stress levels, improves your metabolism, and has a beneficial effect on your microbiome. Aim for 7-8 hours of sleep most days. Consider taking sleep-inducing inulin powder before bed to help your gut to help you sleep (go to cleverguts.com for more information).

TURMERIC TEA

Add 1/2 tsp ground turmeric (or grated fresh) to a cup of hot water, with 1/2 tsp cinnamon and a squeeze of lemon, for a light, nutritious drink or a tangy, aromatic digestif to be sipped after a meal. Just remember to keep stirring the brew as some of the spices slowly sink to the bottom of the cup.

Reduce stress—easier said than done, but we know that chronic pressure and anxiety wreak havoc on your stress hormones, mood, and immune system. The stress hormone cortisol, for example, increases blood sugar and promotes the storage of unhealthy abdominal fat. These hormones are also likely to have an adverse effect on your metabolism, eating patterns, gut bacteria, and, most importantly, on how you feel about yourself. A vicious cycle of low mood, less motivation, and comfort eating may follow. Try to accept things you can't change and deal with things you can. Make some changes, even small ones (though perhaps not all at once!). Mindfulness is an excellent evidence-based way to de-stress and to reduce rumination and the tendency to get stuck in a loop, preoccupied with seemingly insoluble issues.

Practice mindful eating—sit down at a table to eat, and be present in the moment so you are able to focus on what you are eating, to taste it, to savor it. Become aware of the flavor and texture. Is it slightly bitter? Can you taste sweetness or a hint of sour? Or both? Celebrate and enjoy your food. The more interesting and varied, the better for both you and your microbiome. By contrast, if you eat in front of the TV, you probably won't notice any of these satisfying experiences and are likely to eat more in the process. Having your meal at a table can be helpful in other ways, too, particularly if you are eating with others. It can lift your mood and keep you connected. But don't let others push you to eat more than you want, even if it is done as a demonstration of love—learn to say no pleasantly and mean it.

Get more active—we all know that doing exercise is fantastically good for us. It boosts our mood, helps us sleep, cuts our risk of almost every chronic disease (from cancer to dementia), and burns a few calories. There is now good evidence that regular exercise will also improve the quality and diversity of your microbiome. Ideally you should do a mix of exercises that build muscle strength and aerobic fitness.

To keep his muscles in shape Michael likes (well, perhaps not "likes") to do a mix of push-ups, squats, and sit-ups most mornings. For his heart and lungs he takes the dog for the occasional run and cycles where he can, incorporating high-intensity bursts. I try to run for 20 minutes 3 times a week when I can, adding short high-intensity bursts up hills, as well as practice yoga (which incidentally has recently been found to improve gut health, too). The important thing is to push yourself so your heart rate goes up.

If you are not able to commit to specific exercises, you can do yourself a huge amount of good simply by getting outside and moving more. Get your hands dirty, whether in the garden or the park, to get more bugs in your life!

Before You Start

If you have any significant medical problems or very troublesome gut symptoms, we recommend you consult a health professional first. There may be medical reasons for your symptoms that need checking first, such as undiagnosed celiac disease, which can cause low-grade symptoms or even no symptoms at all, but can still lead to significant complications. Other conditions such as inflammatory bowel disease may require further investigation or management. It is important to rule out other potentially significant causes of your symptoms before embarking on dietary changes. It may help to do the program with professional support. If you are underweight, suspect you have a food allergy, have other significant medical problems, or are frail or unwell, we would not advise embarking on this program.

Seek urgent medical advice if you: are passing blood and/or mucus; have severe and/or persistent abdominal pain; experience unexplained, unplanned weight loss or loss of appetite; have a recent change in bowel habit; suffer from anemia or a deficiency in important vitamins or nutrients; have persistent diarrhea and/or vomiting.

Fortunately, food allergies are relatively uncommon. But if you suspect you have one, it is very important that you see your doctor and get tested as it could be life-threatening. Symptoms normally occur within minutes of being in contact with or eating the relevant substance. The typical reaction might involve a blotchy red rash, which is raised and itchy. There may be vomiting and/or severe gut symptoms such as diarrhea; respiratory symptoms resulting in wheezing and difficulty breathing; itching or swelling of the lips, tongue, and palate; or, very rarely, sudden collapse. Once your health professional has helped identify the food substance, you can take measures to avoid it and, if needed, keep emergency medication on hand.

An allergy is different from a food intolerance, which is a nonallergic hypersensitivity, and is much more common. With an intolerance, the onset tends to be delayed by hours, not minutes, and the symptoms are more variable. If you find yourself excluding food, or food groups for a long period of time, we recommend that you consult a professional to ensure that the full clinical picture is considered and that you are getting a healthy balanced diet.

Rebooting Your Biome
with Phases 1 and 2

Most people who pursue the Clever Gut Diet will be doing so to benefit from its general health improvements—a happier, stronger gut and metabolism, as well as weight loss, a reduction in blood sugar, and just feeling better about themselves. However, for those who have gut- and health-related issues that are possibly due to a food sensitivity or intolerance, we would suggest you also try Michael's 2-phase program (see *The Clever Gut Diet*) to reboot your biome.

We would strongly advise that for at least three days beforehand you keep a food diary in which you record the foods eaten and your responses to them. This may be useful if you decide to see a professional about your symptoms. To download our Clever Gut Daily Food and Symptoms Diary, go to cleverguts.com/reboot-your-biome/.

A word on **FODMAPs** (Fermentable Oligosaccharides, Disaccharides, Monosaccharides, and Polyols)—these are a group of poorly absorbed carbohydrates that are found in certain fruits and vegetables. In some people with gut problems, like IBS, these foods get fermented in the bowel, producing more gas, and distension. They can also draw extra fluid into the bowel, causing diarrhea. Although many of these substances are good for a healthy bowel and help feed the microbiome, they may need to be reduced or avoided for IBS and in Phase 1 of the program. The Clever Gut Diet is not specifically a low FODMAP diet, but where possible we have highlighted foods that might exacerbate symptoms of IBS. See cleverguts.com for more information.

. . . and **nightshade vegetables.** On our website, cleverguts.com, people sometimes ask if they should avoid this group of vegetables, of which there are many, including tomatoes, bell peppers, eggplants, and potatoes. They are the edible parts of flowering plants that belong to the Solanaceae family, and are technically classified as fruit. Some people have found they feel better when they reduce their consumption of these foods or remove them completely on the basis that they may contribute to inflammation and leaky gut. If you suspect a problem, it may be worth excluding them for 2-4 weeks (see opposite) without making other changes. Keep a food diary and then reintroduce them (see page 27). But don't avoid them unless you have reason to believe they are at fault. They are an excellent source of nutrients and fiber and are staple foods that have been eaten around the world for millennia.

Phase 1—Removal and Repair

This phase is to give your gut lining a chance to recover, and you should keep to it for about four weeks. The recipes—marked as "**good for Phase 1**"— are specially created for gentle repair and nourishment of the gut. They involve foods which are either low in dairy or dairy-free, low in gluten or gluten-free; and also low in the types of vegetables and beans that are particularly high in fiber and are not digested well by some people (they end up becoming fermented further down the bowel, causing gas, pain, and bloating). This phase does not contain significant amounts of fermented foods either.

If you are looking to test or confirm specific food intolerances, we would recommend you remove no more than one or two foods at a time, and ideally that you do not remove whole food groups. Common culprits implicated in gut problems include gluten, dairy, eggs, soy, and coffee. You can, if necessary, repeat the process at a later date with other suspected foods.

Aim to significantly reduce or ideally avoid:

- Gluten and refined grains
- Dairy products, particularly milk
- Beans, as the lectin in these can cause bloating (though these can be reintroduced after two weeks for vegetarians to maintain protein intake)
- Very fibrous vegetables containing lots of insoluble fiber, such as kale stalks or string beans
- Alcohol and desserts (sorry)

Do include plenty of:

- Non-fibrous, plant-based foods, enough to fill over half your plate, aiming for at least seven portions of vegetables and fruit a day, mainly made up of vegetables—and make them colorful, too
- Good-quality proteins, to aid repair of the gut lining—aim for at least 45-60g a day
- Bitter greens and citrus salads to boost digestion before a meal
- Nondairy fats, such as olive oil and coconut oil, as well as avocados, nuts, and seeds

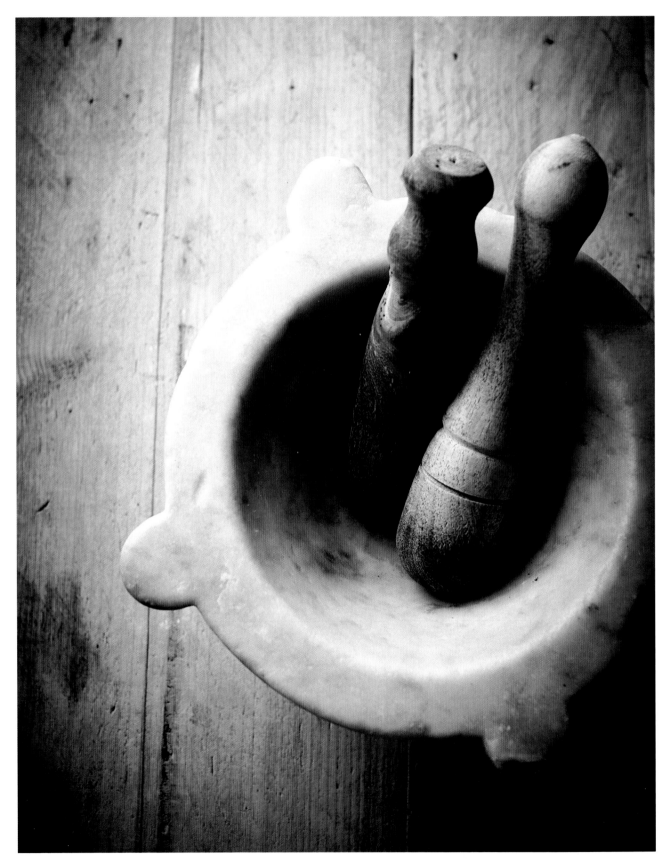

Phase 2—Reintroduction and Recovery

In this phase, you reintroduce variety, more fiber, as well as pre- and probiotics. When you move on to Phase 2, you can choose any recipe in the book.

Increasing prebiotic foods

Prebiotics feed the good microbes (the fertilizer). The following foods are rich in prebiotics so we've included them in our recipes:

- Jerusalem artichokes, onions, leeks, garlic, fennel, asparagus, apples, bok choy
- Beans, lentils, and peas

Increasing probiotics

These are the foods that help top up the good microbes (the seeds). Start with small portions at first so your gut gets used to them:

- Fermented vegetables such as sauerkraut (page 185)
- Active yogurt
- Kefir milk (page 190)
- Cheeses
- Kombucha to drink (page 180)

Reintroducing excluded foods

Try one food at a time, over three days. Eat a normal portion of the suspected food and if symptoms return over the next few days, withdraw that food. Allow a few days' recovery before reintroducing another food. Use the Food and Symptoms Diary (download from cleverguts.com) to monitor your response. In the case of dairy products, you should try full-fat active yogurt first, as this is usually best tolerated, then cheese and butter and milk last of all. If you have excluded all gluten, start with grains that contain relatively little gluten, such as rye or spelt. Sourdough breads (page 198) are easier to digest as the fermentation process breaks down much of the gluten. Then you can move on to a small amount of wheat, again over a few days.

Clever Gut Pantry

Before considering which exciting new ingredients to add to your pantry, we would recommend you do a quick clear-out, removing sugary processed and starchy temptations from your kitchen first—particularly if they are lurking enticingly at the front of your cupboards or on the counter. We don't by any means suggest that you buy all of the items listed below—this is meant to be an inspirational checklist. Buy according to the recipes that appeal to you in general, and remember the Clever Gut mantra: The greater variety of food you eat, the happier and healthier your microbiome will be. To make it easier we have shown the most commonly used ingredients in bold.

SPICES

Black peppercorns
Cardamom pods
Cayenne pepper
Cinnamon, ground
Coriander, ground
**Cumin, seeds
  and ground**
Curry powder
Ginger, ground
Maldon sea salt
Mustard seeds
Nutmeg
Paprika
Pumpkin pie spice
Red pepper flakes
Turmeric, ground
Vanilla extract

HERBS
(Fresh where possible)

Bay leaves
Chives
Dill
Oregano
Parsley
Tarragon
Thyme

FLOURS AND BAKING

Baking powder
Baking soda
Buckwheat flour
Chickpea flour (besan)
Ground almonds
Rye flour
Spelt flour
Whole wheat flour
Xanthan gum

GRAINS, BEANS, AND PASTA

Black beans, canned
Borlotti beans, canned
Brown rice
Bulgur wheat
Butter beans, canned
Cannellini beans, canned
Chickpeas, canned
Green lentils, canned
Green-pea pasta shapes
Kidney beans, canned
Puy lentils, cooked,
  vacuum-packed
Quinoa
Red lentils, dried
Red rice
Rolled oats
Soba noodles

OILS AND VINEGARS

Balsamic vinegar
Coconut oil
Extra-virgin olive oil
Light olive oil
Olive oil
Rapeseed oil
Raw, unfiltered apple cider vinegar
Rice wine vinegar
Sesame oil

FLAVORINGS, SAUCES, SWEETENERS, AND PASTES

Basil pesto
Cacao powder
Dark chocolate (70%)
Desiccated coconut
Fresh ginger
Garlic
Harissa paste
Honey
Maple syrup
Mirin
Miso
Mustard, Dijon and whole grain
Nori seaweed
Organic tea (for kombucha)
Tabasco
Tahini
Tamari
Thai fish sauce
Tomato puree
Worcestershire sauce
Yeast extract

CANNED OR BOTTLED FOODS

Anchovies
Artichoke hearts
Capers
Coconut cream
Coconut milk
Crab
Jalapeño peppers
Nondairy milks (soy, almond)
Nut butters (cashew, almond)
Olives
Pureed pumpkin
Roasted red peppers
Sardines
Soy cream
Tomatoes
Tuna

NUTS AND SEEDS

Almonds, slivered and blanched
Brazil nuts
Cashews
Chia seeds
Flaxseed, ground
Hazelnuts
Pecans
Pine nuts
Pistachios
Pumpkin seeds
Sesame seeds
Sunflower seeds
Walnuts

DRIED FRUIT

Apricots
Cranberries
Dates
Raisins

IN THE FRIDGE

Butter
Buttermilk
Cheese (Parmesan, vegan Parmesan, sharp Cheddar, feta, halloumi)
Cream cheese
Crème fraîche
Eggs, free-range
Full-fat active Greek-style yogurt
Kefir
Lemons
Limes
Raspberries, blueberries, strawberries

IN THE FREEZER

Baby peas
Berries
Chicken breasts
Edamame
Fish (salmon, cod, etc.)
Shrimp
Spinach

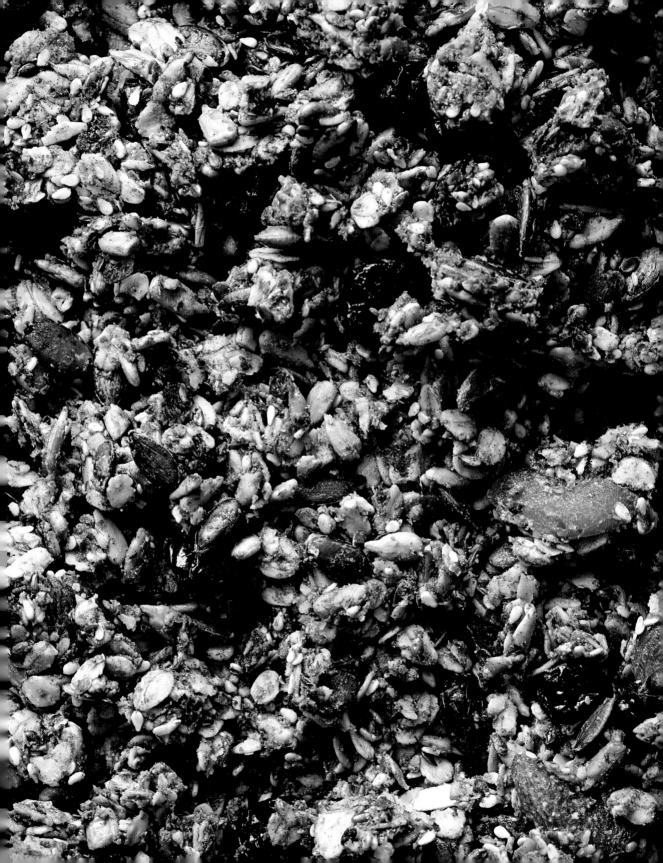

BREAKFAST

A good breakfast, eaten
mindfully, while seated,
is the best way to start
the day.

Yogurt

Full-fat active yogurt ticks all the Mediterranean-style healthy-eating boxes. The natural fats in it have little impact on cardiovascular disease—they may even have a beneficial effect—and its live microorganisms feed the good bacteria in your gut. If you make your own yogurt, then even better—you know it's going to be full of lovely live cultures. We recommend Greek-style yogurt as the straining process increases the protein and nutrient content. But there are good nondairy equivalents available, too.

Yogurt with Granola and Diced Pear

We particularly enjoy this combination, which also makes an easy dessert shared between two.

Serves 1

1 small pear, cored and diced

1 cup full-fat active Greek-style yogurt (or non-dairy equivalent)

2 tbsp Healthy Homemade Granola (page 34)

• DAIRY-FREE OPTION

• GLUTEN-FREE

• GOOD FOR PHASE 1

1. Place the diced pear in a jar or bowl.

2. Add the yogurt and sprinkle the granola on top. Easy.

Tip: Those of you on Phase 2 can try substituting kefir for the yogurt; it has a delicious tartness and delivers even more good probiotics to your microbiome. To make your own kefir, see page 190. Add a drizzle of maple syrup if you find the kefir too sour, or add some diced strawberries.

440 CALORIES

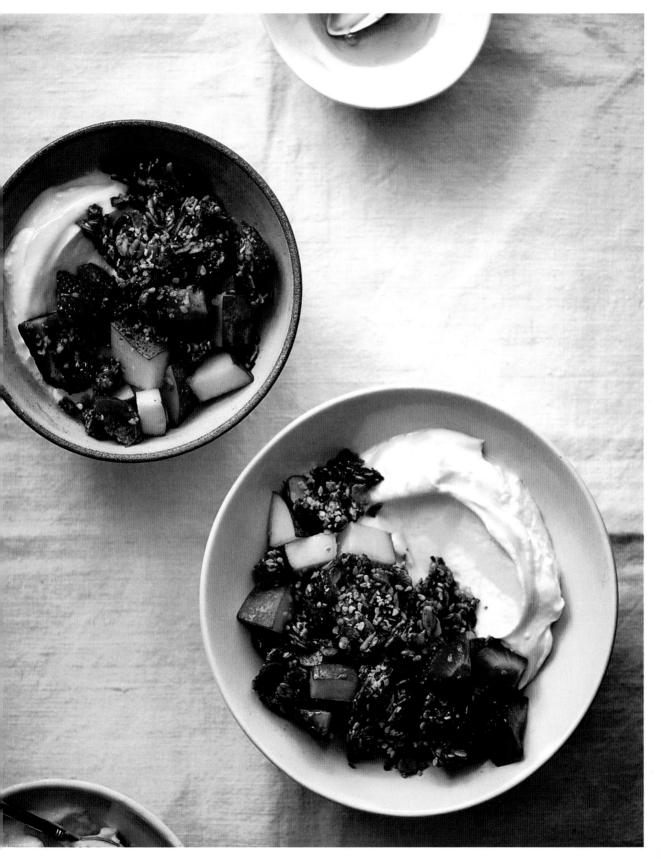

Healthy Homemade Granola

This crunchy granola is full of toasted nutty flavors. If you make it yourself you know it's gluten-free and that it's also likely to be much lower in sugar than most supermarket versions. Seeds, nuts, and unprocessed oats are absorbed slowly in the gut as they are made of complex carbohydrates containing lots of fiber. And your microbiome will thrive on the fiber, too.

Makes 12 servings

Scant ½ cup coconut oil, melted

15 large soft dates, finely chopped

1 tsp salt

2 tsp vanilla extract

1 egg white, to bind

2½ cups gluten-free rolled oats

1½ cups mixed seeds (such as sunflower, sesame, and pumpkin) and nuts (such as almonds, cashews, or pistachios)

¾ cup ground flaxseeds

⅔ cup dried fruit, such as cranberries, raisins, or diced apricots

• DAIRY-FREE
• GLUTEN-FREE
• GOOD FOR PHASE 1

1. Preheat the oven to 250°F. Blitz the coconut oil, dates, salt, vanilla, and egg white in a food processor or with a hand blender to form a rough paste.

2. Put the oats, seeds and nuts, flaxseeds, and dried fruit in a medium bowl and pour in the date mixture, working it evenly into the oats with a wooden spoon.

3. Scatter the mixture in the bottom of a medium baking sheet lined with parchment paper and bake for 25-30 minutes. Then turn the oven off and leave it to crisp up for an hour or two, or even overnight, before breaking it up into small clusters. It can be stored in an airtight jar for up to a month, or in the freezer for several months.

Tip: 1-2 tbsp water can be used instead of the egg white.

340 CALORIES

Yogurt with Chia Jam and Toasted Pistachios

Abandon those low-fat sugary yogurts for the real thing—thick and creamy full-fat yogurt is back on the menu as a staple in a healthy diet. The chia jam and toasted nuts here will give you all the sweetness you need.

Serves 1

1 tbsp Strawberry Chia Jam
   (page 208)
1 cup full-fat active Greek-
   style yogurt (or non-
   dairy equivalent)
Handful of berries, such
   as raspberries,
   strawberries, or
   blueberries
1 tbsp toasted nuts, such
   as pistachios or almonds

•DAIRY-FREE OPTION
•GLUTEN-FREE
•GOOD FOR PHASE 1

1. Spoon the chia jam into a glass or small jar.

2. Dollop the yogurt on top, and then sprinkle with the berries and nuts.

230 CALORIES

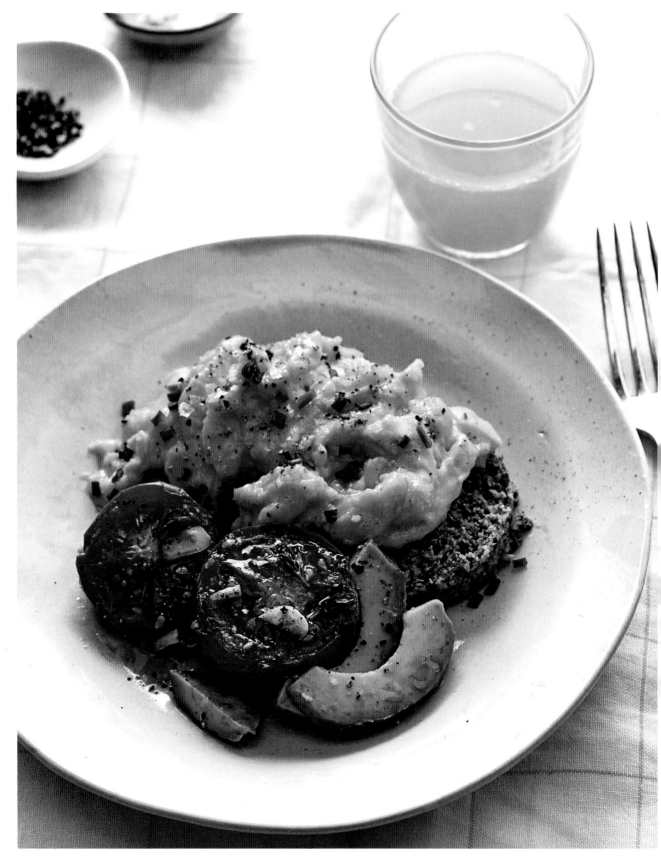

Eggs

Michael and I love eggs. Fears that they raise cholesterol are unfounded. Embrace them. Enjoy them. See how good you feel going to work on an egg.

Simple Creamy Scrambled Eggs

Serves 1

2 eggs

Small pat of butter or
  drizzle of oil

•DAIRY-FREE OPTION

•GLUTEN-FREE

•GOOD FOR PHASE 1

1. Whisk the eggs with a fork in a bowl. In a small nonstick pan, melt the butter over low heat, without allowing it to brown. Pour in the eggs and stir gently with a wooden spoon for 1-2 minutes.

2. Remove the eggs from the heat when they start to thicken but are still a bit runny in places. Transfer them immediately to the plate. Scatter some sea salt and black pepper (or a pinch of red pepper flakes) on top. You can jazz them up with a few fresh herbs, such as chopped chives.

190 CALORIES

With smoked salmon: Top with scant 2 ounces smoked salmon, a squeeze of lemon, and ground black pepper to taste (add 90 calories).

With leafy greens and Parmesan: Add a cup of cooked leftover greens and ¼ cup grated Parmesan (or vegan Parmesan) as you scramble the eggs (add 100 calories).

With cremini mushrooms: Fry the mushrooms in oil or butter for 4-5 minutes. Season, scatter with chopped parsley, and serve alongside the scrambled eggs (add 60 calories, plus another 60 calories if you use ½ tbsp oil for frying).

On a slice of toast: Try your scrambled eggs on a slice of toasted Mug Bread (page 194; see pic, *left*) or No-Knead Sourdough (page 198) with butter (add 300 calories).

Turmeric Spiced Omelet with Seaweed

Give your omelet an extra kick with this spiced coconut mixture, which contains two fabulously gut-friendly ingredients, turmeric and seaweed.

Serves 2

Small pat of butter
  or drizzle of oil

4 medium mushrooms,
  finely chopped

4 eggs

1 tbsp Dry Coconut Sambal
  (page 120)

•DAIRY-FREE OPTION

•GLUTEN-FREE

•GOOD FOR PHASE 1

1. Heat the butter in a small frying pan and sauté the mushrooms for about 5 minutes, or until they are soft.

2. Beat the eggs in a bowl and pour them into the pan. Lower the heat, scatter the coconut sambal on top, and cook until the bottom of the omelet is starting to firm up but the top is still moist. Season with black pepper. Fold the omelet over, cut it in half, and serve immediately.

Tip: Ground black pepper massively enhances the benefit of turmeric.

270 CALORIES

Mushroom Omelet with Red Sauerkraut

Sauerkraut works well added to an omelet, providing a salty, tangy crunch and lots of good bugs for your microbiome.

Serves 1

Small pat of butter
  or drizzle of oil

2 medium cremini
  mushrooms, finely diced

2 eggs

1 tbsp Red Cabbage
  Sauerkraut (page 185)

•DAIRY-FREE OPTION

•GLUTEN-FREE

1. Heat the butter in a small frying pan and sauté the mushrooms for about 5 minutes, or until they are soft.

2. Beat the eggs in a bowl and pour them into the pan. Lower the heat and cook until the bottom of the omelet is starting to firm up but the top is still moist. Fold the omelet over and transfer it to a plate. Spread the sauerkraut on top, and season with black pepper.

Tip: For Phase 1, skip the sauerkraut.

220 CALORIES

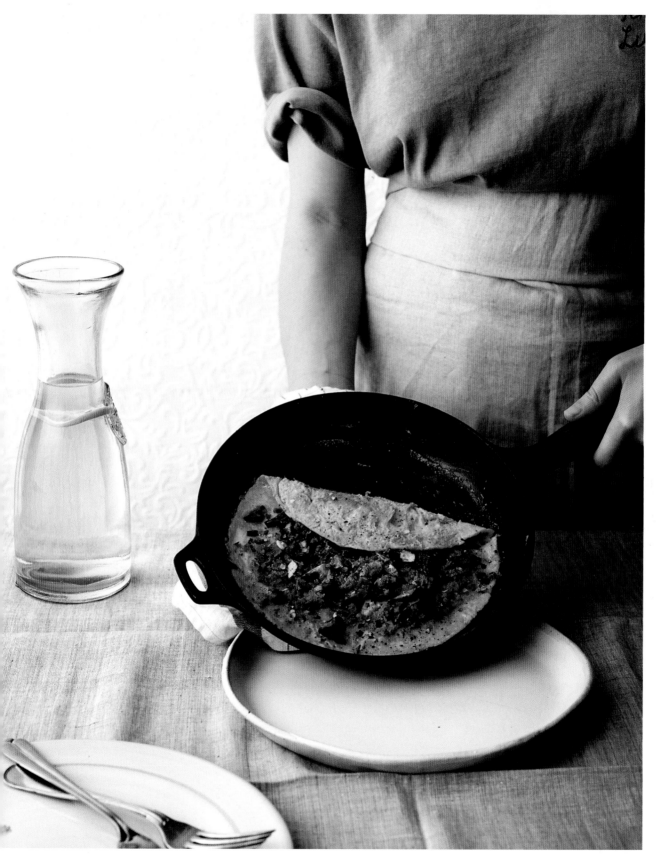

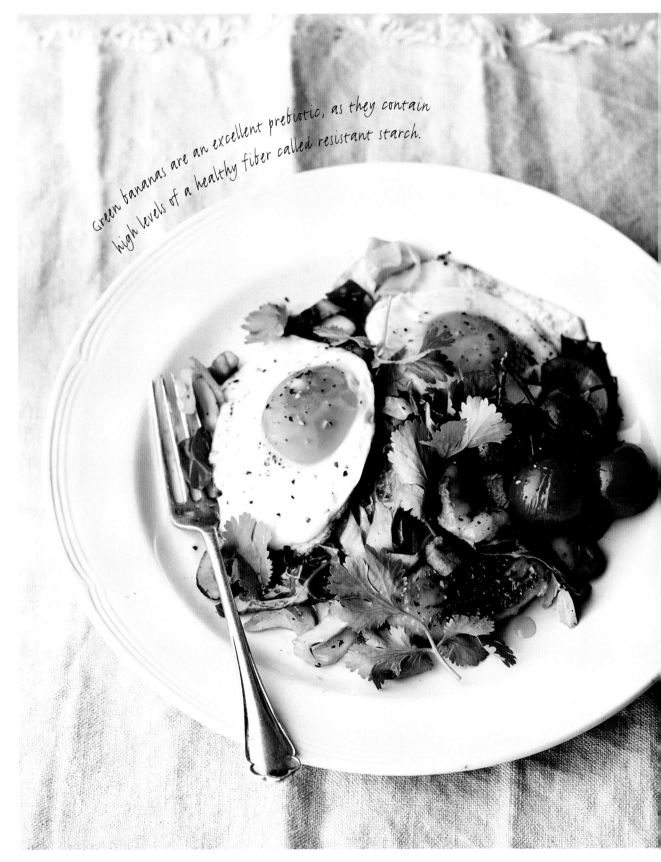

Green bananas are an excellent prebiotic, as they contain high levels of a healthy fiber called resistant starch.

Full English Breakfast with Green Bananas

Our kids have turned the breakfast "fry-up" into a well-honed art form, cooked with more enthusiasm than almost any other meal. Try this gut-friendly version, made with green bananas, which have an astonishing 70-80% resistant starch. (Sadly this drops to only 1% in ripe bananas as the starch gets converted into simple sugars—sucrose, glucose, and fructose.) I got to love fried green bananas after eating them for breakfast every day while working on a medical project in the Amazon jungle.

Serves 2

2 oz pancetta cubes
    or diced bacon
2-3 tbsp olive oil
4 oz mushrooms, sliced
1 large green banana,
    halved lengthwise
2 eggs
5 oz cooked cabbage or
    kale, chopped and tough
    stalks removed (leftover
    greens are ideal)
5 oz small plum tomatoes,
    halved
½ tsp ground nutmeg

•DAIRY-FREE
•GLUTEN-FREE
•GOOD FOR PHASE 1

1. Place the pancetta in a small frying pan over medium heat and fry it for about 5 minutes, or until it is brown and crispy, then set it aside.

2. Pour the oil into another, larger frying pan and fry the mushrooms and banana over medium heat. Season with salt and pepper. Clear a space in the middle of the pan, add a little more oil if necessary, and crack in the eggs.

3. Season the greens and add them to the pan with the tomatoes and nutmeg, then scatter the pancetta on top. Cook everything for a couple more minutes—the egg yolk should still be a bit runny. Serve on warm plates.

Tip: Keep the green banana in the fridge so it does not ripen and convert to sugars.

440 CALORIES

Oatmeal

Toss those processed breakfast cereals, most of which are stuffed with hidden sugars. That also includes instant oatmeal, which contains little of the complex carbohydrates or fiber needed by your microbiome. Our porridge recipes use whole oats, which are only minimally processed and still contain the nutritious inner kernel of the oats, along with plenty of fiber and nutrients to keep you going well into the day.

Coconut Oatmeal with Pecans and Pear

A creamy, nutty oatmeal laced with sweet juicy pear.

Serves 2
⅔ cup rolled oats (or gluten-free)
¾ cup coconut milk
½ tsp ground cinnamon
¼ tsp ground nutmeg
Pinch of salt
2 tbsp coarsely chopped pecans
½ pear, cored and diced

•DAIRY-FREE
•GLUTEN-FREE OPTION
•GOOD FOR PHASE 1

1. Place the oats, coconut milk, spices, salt, and pecans in a small pan and bring it to a simmer. Cook for 10-12 minutes, stirring frequently, until the mixture is thick and creamy.

2. Pour it into 2 bowls, scatter the diced pear on top, and dig in. A teaspoonful of honey won't harm, but it's just as good without.

370 CALORIES

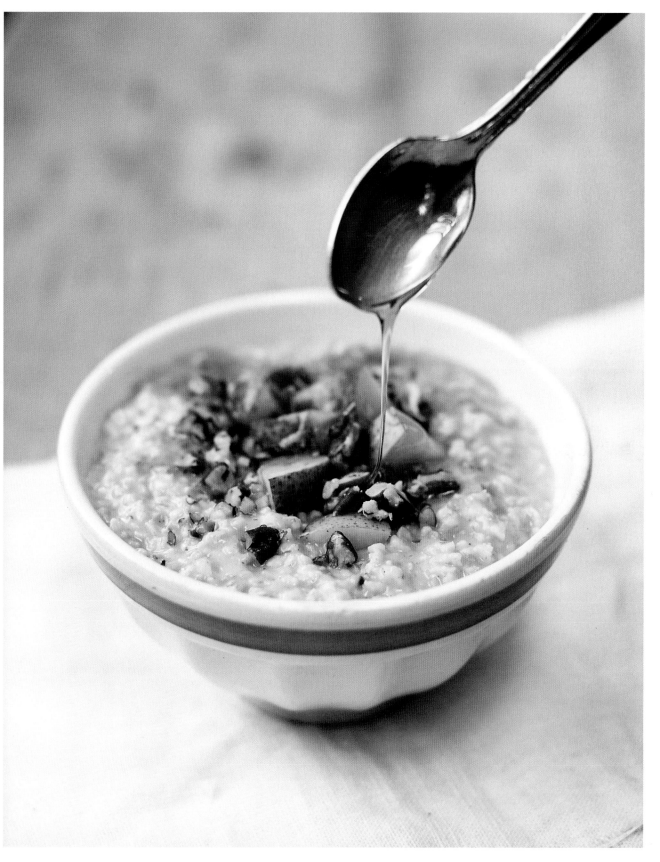

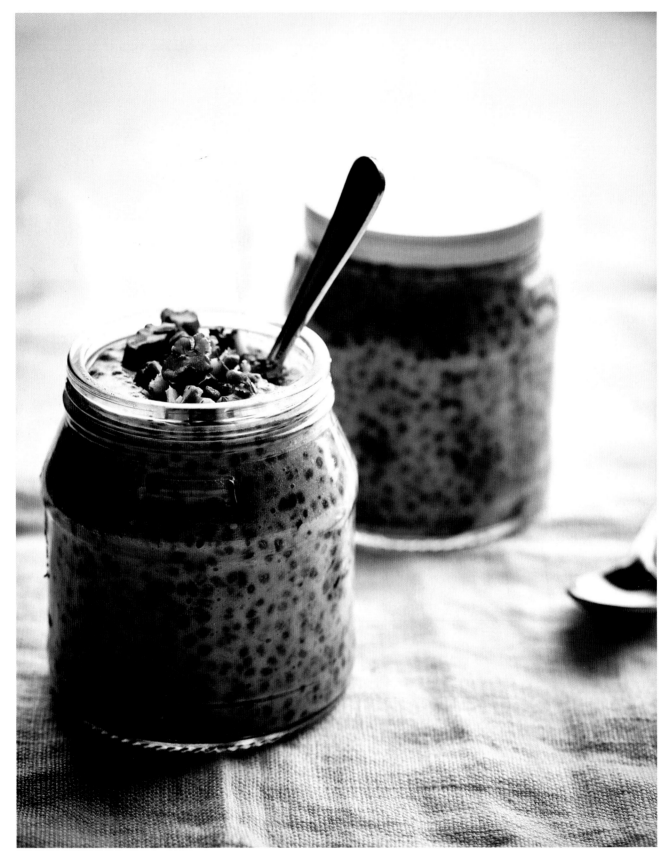

Blueberry Chia Pots

Serves 2

1 (14-oz) can coconut milk

3 tbsp chia seeds

1 tsp vanilla extract

1 tsp ground nutmeg

Juice of 1 large lemon

1½ cups blueberries

3 tbsp pecans, coarsely
  chopped

•DAIRY-FREE

•GLUTEN-FREE

•GOOD FOR PHASE 1

1. With a food processor or hand blender, blitz the coconut milk, chia, vanilla, and nutmeg for about 1 minute, or until you have a smooth creamy mixture. Add the lemon juice and blueberries and pulse briefly—you want to retain some texture.

2. Spoon the mixture into pots or bowls and leave it to thicken in the fridge overnight, or for at least 30 minutes.

3. When you are ready to eat it, scatter the pecans on top.

Tip: This also makes a great dessert—divide it into 4 portions and halve the calorie count.

590 CALORIES

Bircher Muesli with Kefir

Serves 4

2½ cups rolled oats

⅓ cup cashews

¼ cup sesame seeds

2 tbsp pumpkin seeds

⅓ cup desiccated coconut

¼ cup dried cranberries

1¾ cups almond milk
  (or dairy milk if using)

¾ cup kefir (see page 190)
  or nondairy equivalent

1 cup berries, such as
  blueberries or raspberries

•DAIRY-FREE OPTION

•GOOD FOR PHASE 1

1. Put the oats in a bowl or glass jar with the cashews, sesame and pumpkin seeds, coconut, and cranberries. Stir in the milk and store it in the fridge, covered, overnight. (Soaking muesli helps to break down the cell walls in the seeds, nuts, and fruits, making them easier to digest.)

2. Before serving, stir in the kefir and scatter the berries on top.

Tip: Store it in the fridge or freeze extra portions for another day.

450 CALORIES

Fatty Fish

Fatty fish works wonders in your gut and is one of the best possible sources of omega-3 fatty acids—something we need to eat more of to create a healthy balance with the more readily available omega-6s. Fatty fish helps to keep down blood sugar, too.

Avocado and Smoked Salmon

Simple, high in protein and omega-3s, this is a great breakfast that will keep you full for the rest of the morning.

Serves 2

1 avocado, thinly sliced
6 oz smoked salmon
Juice of ½ lemon

•DAIRY-FREE
•GLUTEN-FREE
•GOOD FOR PHASE 1

1. Divide the avocado between 2 plates, fanning out the slices.

2. Place the salmon on top with a generous squeeze of lemon juice and a grinding of black pepper. Serve immediately.

280 CALORIES

Smoked Mackerel and Kale Kedgeree

So quick to make and so tasty, with turmeric for added flavor and a healthy anti-inflammatory boost.

Serves 4

⅔ cup brown basmati rice

2 tbsp olive oil

1 onion, diced

½ red bell pepper, seeded and diced

1 tsp curry powder

½ tsp turmeric

6 oz cauliflower, broken into florets

2 handfuls of kale, shredded

3 smoked mackerel or smoked trout fillets, skinned and broken into chunks

4 hard-boiled eggs, halved

• DAIRY-FREE

• GLUTEN-FREE

• GOOD FOR PHASE 1

1. Cook the rice according to the package instructions, ideally the night before. Leave it to chill in the fridge.

2. Meanwhile, heat the oil in a large frying pan and sauté the onion and bell pepper for 4-5 minutes. Stir in the spices and cook for another minute, before adding the cauliflower and rice.

3. Cook for 2-3 minutes, stirring occasionally, then add the kale and smoked mackerel and cook for 4-5 minutes longer, until the kale has wilted and the mackerel is heated through.

4. Gently stir the eggs into the kedgeree and season to taste before serving.

540 CALORIES

Clever Smoothies

Nutrient-rich shakes make a great one-stop meal for those who don't feel like eating first thing in the morning or don't have time for breakfast. If you blitz them less, they retain more texture, ensuring that you still get plenty of healthy fiber for those bugs to get their teeth into. The natural fats we have included will help you feel satiated without spiking your blood sugar. They will also improve the absorption of fat-soluble vitamins.

Clever Gut Green Smoothie

A satisfying start to the day, full of green goodness.

Serves 1
4 celery stalks, chopped
Small handful of kale, chopped, tough stalks removed
Large handful of spinach
2 bok choy, green leaves only
½ avocado, sliced
½ cup blueberries
2 tbsp full-fat active Greek-style yogurt (or nondairy equivalent)
1 tbsp olive oil
Handful of ice cubes

•DAIRY-FREE OPTION
•GLUTEN-FREE
•GOOD FOR PHASE 1

1. Place all the ingredients in a blender with ¾ cup water and blitz for 10-20 seconds. The mixture should retain a little texture.

2. Pour it into a jug and store in the fridge. It will keep for up to 24 hours.

Note: If you have IBS you might wish to reduce the amount of celery.

450 CALORIES

These drinks are ideal to keep you going on a fast day—
one serving will provide about half of your daily calorie count,
the rest of which you can make up with a meal.

Dr. Tim's Healthy Gut Smoothie

A thick, fruity smoothie shared by our great friend Tim in Australia, who slimmed back down to the figure he had at medical school by drinking these as part of his 5:2 fast day regimen.

Serves 1

½ avocado, sliced

1 apple, cored and chopped

2 bok choy, green leaves only

1 tbsp olive oil

2 tbsp full-fat active Greek-style yogurt (or nondairy equivalent)

3 tbsp dairy or nondairy milk, such as almond or soy

Large handful of spinach leaves

½ cup frozen strawberries or blueberries

Handful of ice cubes

•DAIRY-FREE OPTION

•GLUTEN-FREE

•GOOD FOR PHASE 1

1. Place all the ingredients in a blender and blitz for 10-20 seconds. The mixture should retain a little texture.

2. Pour it into a jug and store in the fridge. It will keep for up to 24 hours.

520 CALORIES

Creamy Pineapple Smoothie

Pineapple is one of the surprise ingredients of the Clever Gut Diet. Not only is it rich in fiber, it also contains an enzyme called bromelain which helps digestion, particularly of protein, and is thought to have anti-inflammatory properties.

Serves 2

12 oz fresh pineapple, skin
   removed, chopped
⅓ cup cashews
⅓ cup sunflower seeds
¾ cup kefir (see page 190)
   or buttermilk (or
   nondairy equivalent)
½ cup almond milk
Pinch of ground cinnamon

•DAIRY-FREE OPTION
•GLUTEN-FREE
•GOOD FOR PHASE 1

Place all the ingredients in a blender and blitz until you have a fairly smooth mixture. Serve immediately.

Tip: If your blender does not break down nuts or seeds easily, try soaking them in the milk for an hour first.

460 CALORIES

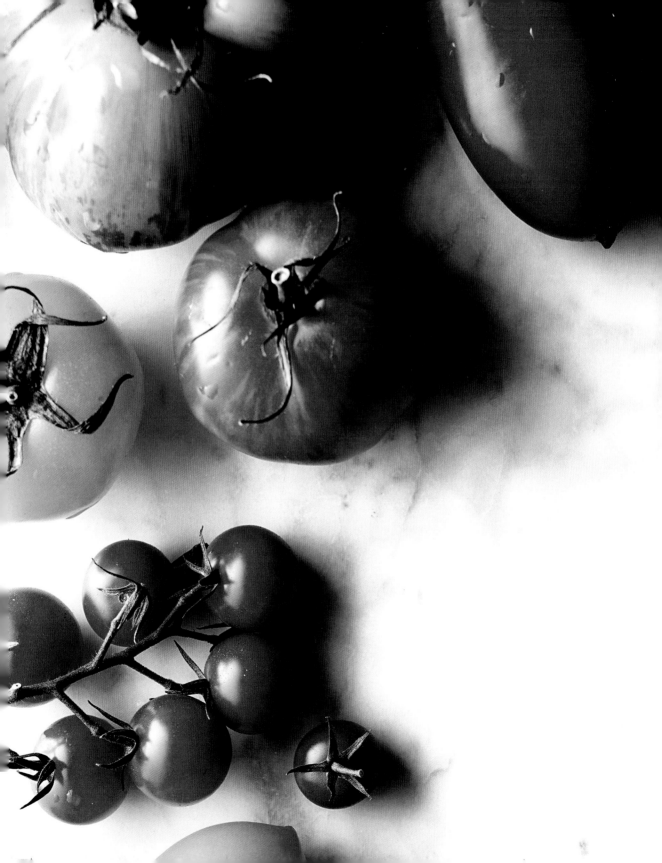

LIGHT MEALS, SOUPS, AND SALADS

Enzyme-stimulating salads, healing
broths, gut-friendly snacks, and a range
of simple, tasty dishes to expand
your daily repertoire and nurture
your good bacteria.

The live bacteria in the buttermilk dressing deliver a boost of probiotics to your gut . . . while the vitamin C in the citrus fruit increases the absorption of iron.

Enzyme-Stimulating Salads

Eating bitter greens (such as arugula, watercress, or spinach) or sharp citrus fruits before or with your meal helps get the digestive process going.

Citrus, Fennel, and Asparagus Salad

Serves 2

8 large asparagus spears

1 large orange, peeled and sliced

1 fennel bulb, halved and thinly sliced

2 handfuls bitter greens

¼ cup Lemony Buttermilk Dressing (page 118)

•GLUTEN-FREE

•GOOD FOR PHASE 1

1. Sear the asparagus on a very hot grill pan for 4-5 minutes, turning frequently. Transfer to a plate and slice each spear in half lengthwise.

2. Place the asparagus and all the other ingredients in a salad bowl and toss them with the dressing.

Tip: To make this salad more substantial you can add 1/4 cup crumbled goat cheese and 1/3 cup toasted hazelnuts (add 250 calories per portion).

100 CALORIES

Blood Orange Salad with Toasted Coriander

Serves 2

1 blood orange, peeled

Small bunch of watercress

½ red onion, thinly sliced

1 tsp coriander seeds

¼ cup olive oil

Juice of ½ lemon

•DAIRY-FREE

•GLUTEN-FREE

•GOOD FOR PHASE 1

1. Break the orange into segments, and place them with the watercress and onion in a salad bowl.

2. Toast and lightly crush the coriander seeds, and whisk them with the oil and lemon juice. Pour the dressing over the salad and toss well before serving.

280 CALORIES

Bitter Greens and Toasted Pine Nut Salad

One of our top ten Clever Gut ingredients, apple cider vinegar has been shown to reduce blood sugar and even encourage weight loss in some individuals. It contains a host of live microbiome-enhancing microorganisms—if left in the cupboard it may grow wispy strands and form a "mother" made up of proteins, enzymes, bacteria, and yeasts, which only enhance the benefits.

Serves 2

3 tbsp olive oil

1 tbsp raw unfiltered apple cider vinegar

2 generous handfuls arugula, watercress, dandelion greens, or baby spinach, or a mixture

1 tbsp Parmesan shavings (or vegan Parmesan)

2 tbsp pine nuts, toasted

• DAIRY-FREE OPTION

• GLUTEN-FREE

• GOOD FOR PHASE 1

1. To make the dressing, whisk the oil and vinegar and season with Maldon sea salt and freshly ground black pepper.

2. Place the salad leaves in a bowl, and toss them with the dressing.

3. Sprinkle the Parmesan shavings and pine nuts on top before serving.

Tip: For a more filling salad add 1¼ oz fresh marinated anchovies, available online and in gourmet supermarkets. They will not only add flavor, but also check off the fatty fish box (add about 35 calories).

260 CALORIES

Cider Vinegar Aperitif

If you don't have time for a salad, you can simply drink a diluted gin-and-tonic sized portion of this before a meal to stimulate digestion.

Serves 1

½-1 tbsp raw unfiltered apple cider vinegar

⅔-¾ cup water

• DAIRY-FREE

• GLUTEN-FREE

Add the vinegar to either warm or cold water. You can make it a bit stronger than this, but don't overdo it; it is not currently recommended to have more than 2 tbsp of vinegar a day.

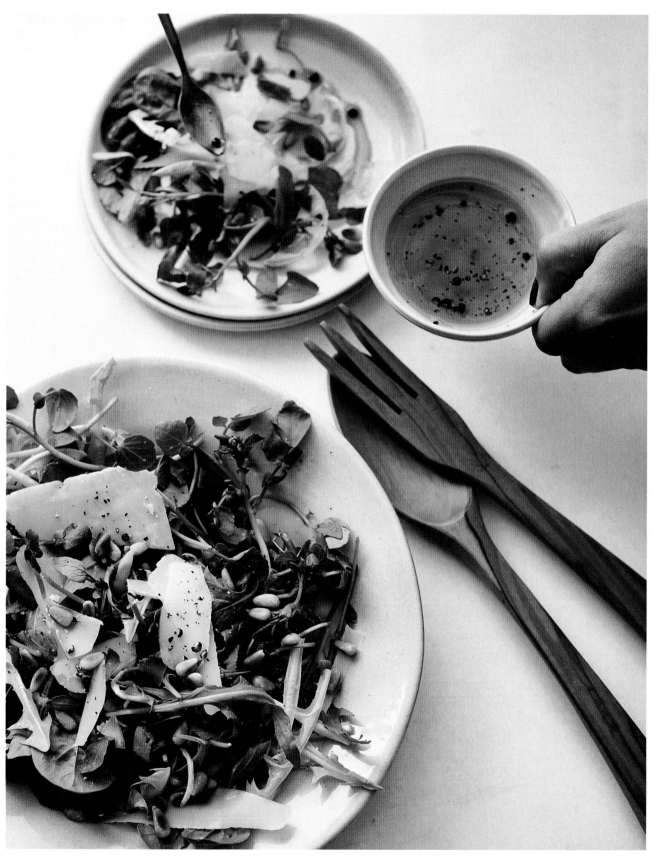

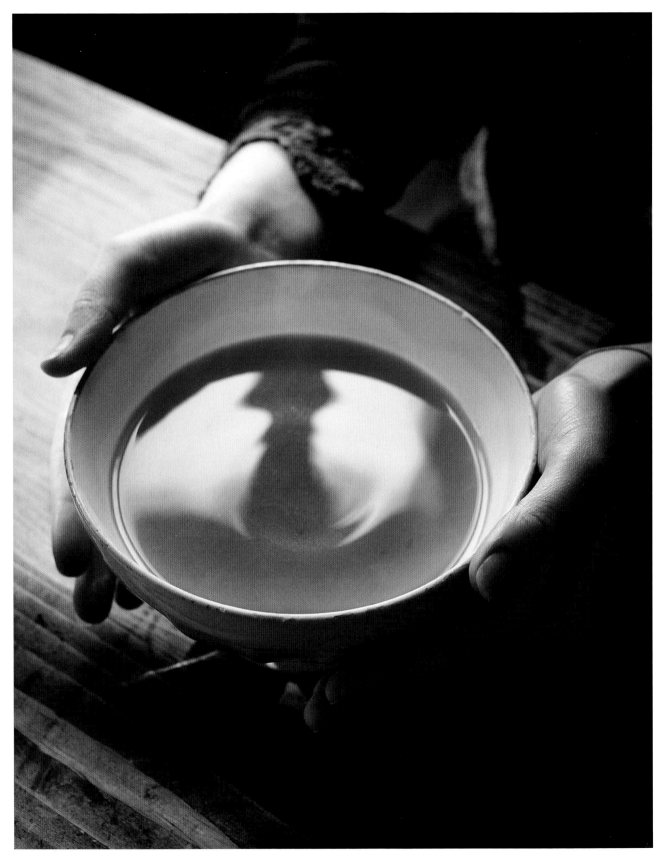

Broths and Soups

Broths, which are slow-cooked to release minerals and nutrients from bones, are wonderfully nourishing for the gut. Soup, meanwhile, has the magical ability to reduce blood sugar spikes that would be caused by eating the individual ingredients separately, offering maximum nutrition while keeping you full for longer. This is because the food is emulsified and therefore digested more slowly. A bowl of steaming soup enhances life.

Healing Chicken Bone Broth

A classic medicinal food used all over the world to soothe troubled guts and aid recovery after illness. A perfect way to use up leftover chicken bones.

Makes about 2 quarts, serves 8

3 tbsp olive oil
4 celery stalks, chopped
2 small onions, chopped
2 leeks, trimmed
1 large garlic clove, halved
2 carrots, chopped
2¼ lb chicken wings and/or chicken carcasses
1 tbsp raw unfiltered apple cider vinegar
2 bay leaves
1 bouquet garni
Handful of parsley sprigs
6-8 black peppercorns

•DAIRY-FREE
•GLUTEN-FREE
•GOOD FOR PHASE 1

1. Heat the oil in a stockpot and sauté the celery, onions, and leeks for 5-7 minutes. Add the garlic, carrots, chicken, vinegar, bay leaves, bouquet garni, parsley, and peppercorns.

2. Add 2-2½ quarts water and bring to a simmer. Cover and cook for at least 3 hours, ideally for 5-6 hours to get the most nutrients from the bones. Check occasionally to ensure that it has not dried out, topping off with water if needed and skimming any scum from the surface.

3. Place a sieve over a large bowl and pour the stock through it, allowing it to drip for 15 minutes. For a thicker, tastier broth you can gently press the soft vegetables through the sieve with a spoon. Use the broth immediately or let it cool, then ladle into containers and keep in the fridge for up to 5 days. It can also be frozen.

40 CALORIES

Gut-Soothing Vegetable Bouillon

This classic vegetable stock makes an excellent clear soup, and can also be used as a tasty and nutritious base for all sorts of recipes, from stews or casseroles to sauces. It can be kept in the fridge for five days or frozen in portions ready to use when needed.

Makes about 4 cups, serves 4

2 tbsp olive oil

1 large onion, halved and coarsely chopped

4 oz carrots, coarsely chopped

4 oz leeks, trimmed and cut into 1- to 1½-inch pieces

4 oz celery, cut into 1- to 1½-inch pieces

Large handful of fresh parsley, including stalks

2 garlic cloves

3 bay leaves

8-10 black peppercorns

1 tbsp Maldon sea salt

•DAIRY-FREE

•GLUTEN-FREE

•GOOD FOR PHASE 1

1. Heat the oil in a large pan and sauté the onion gently for 4-5 minutes, or until it is soft. Add the remaining ingredients, along with 4-6 cups water and bring to a boil. Cover the pan, reduce the heat, and allow it to simmer for 1-1½ hours.

2. Place a sieve over a large bowl and pour the stock through it. To boost the flavor and get a thicker broth, gently press the soft vegetables through the sieve with a spoon.

3. The stock can be stored in the fridge for up to 5 days, or in the freezer.

20 CALORIES

Quick Seaweed Miso Soup

Ideal for a 5:2 fast day, this excellent seaweed broth was suggested by Fatrabbit, a member of the Clever Guts Forum, as a low-calorie drink that is surprisingly filling and packed with nutrients. Miso is a traditional Japanese seasoning produced by fermenting soybeans with salt and koji, a yeast fermentation starter, and sometimes with rice, barley, or other ingredients. It may not be suitable if you are very gluten-sensitive as it can contain small amounts of gluten; however, gluten-free equivalents are available.

Serves 1

1 tbsp chopped dried
   seaweed (such as nori)

1 tsp miso

•DAIRY-FREE
•GLUTEN-FREE OPTION

Place the seaweed and miso in a mug and top up with boiling water. Leave it to stand for 1-2 minutes before drinking it.

15 CALORIES

Spicy Lentil and Tomato Soup

This comforting and fiber-rich soup is easily made using Vegetable-Rich Tomato Sauce (page 168) and Gut-Soothing Vegetable Bouillon (page 60). Lentils are added for extra protein and fiber.

Serves 2

1⅓ cups Vegetable-Rich
   Tomato Sauce (page 168)
¼ cup red lentils
2 cups Gut-Soothing
   Vegetable Bouillon
   (page 60) or stock of
   your choice
¼ tsp red pepper flakes
   (optional)
Small handful of fresh
   cilantro, chopped

•DAIRY-FREE
•GLUTEN-FREE

1. Place the tomato sauce, lentils, vegetable bouillon, and red pepper flakes in a medium pan and bring to a simmer. Cook for 30 minutes, or until the lentils are soft.

2. Scatter the cilantro on top just before serving.

Tip: To make this soup more filling, drizzle with 1/2 tbsp extra-virgin olive oil (add 60 calories), add 1/4 cup grated cheese (add 160 calories), scatter 1/2 tbsp toasted seeds on top (add 60 calories), or add 1 tbsp chopped fried chorizo (add 90 calories).

160 CALORIES

Green Gazpacho with Seaweed

A green, gut-friendly chilled soup with seaweed has a subtle savory flavor along with some extra health-boosting omega-3s.

Serves 2

2½ cups watercress or baby spinach leaves
½ cucumber, coarsely chopped
2 tomatoes, halved
½ green chile, seeded and coarsely chopped
1 garlic clove, chopped
2 large nori seaweed sheets, sliced (optional)
2 spring onions, trimmed and coarsely chopped
1 avocado, halved
3 tbsp extra-virgin olive oil, plus more for drizzling
1 tbsp raw unfiltered apple cider vinegar
Small handful of fresh mint and parsley leaves, coarsely chopped

•DAIRY-FREE
•GLUTEN-FREE
•GOOD FOR PHASE 1

1. Place the watercress, cucumber, tomatoes, chile, garlic, nori, onions, and avocado in a food processor and blend until everything has broken down a little.

2. Add the oil and vinegar and pulse again. Slowly pour in ⅔-1 cup cold water until you reach your desired consistency. Season well to taste.

3. Serve the gazpacho in bowls with a drizzle of oil, a few ice cubes, and a sprinkling of mint and parsley.

380 CALORIES

Pink Celeriac and Beet Soup

Knobbly and a bit awkward to handle, celeriac needs only the minimum of peeling, as most of the nutrients are concentrated just beneath the skin. Like beets, celeriac is full of the kind of complex carbohydrates loved by your gut biome. The delicate flavors of the two root vegetables combine beautifully here to make a creamy and filling soup.

Serves 4

3 tbsp olive oil

1 small onion, chopped

¾ lb beets, peeled and chopped into ¾-inch cubes

1¾ lb celeriac, peeled and chopped into ¾-inch cubes

1 inch fresh ginger, diced

Juice of ½ lemon

¼-½ tsp red pepper flakes

4 cups vegetable stock, or Gut-Soothing Vegetable Bouillon (page 60)

Grated cheese or toasted nuts, for serving (optional)

•DAIRY-FREE

•GLUTEN-FREE

•GOOD FOR PHASE 1

1. Heat the oil in a medium pan and sauté the onion for 5 minutes, or until it has softened.

2. Add the beets, celeriac, ginger, lemon juice, and red pepper flakes, then pour in the stock. Bring to a boil and cook, covered, for about 20 minutes, or until the vegetables are tender.

3. Puree the soup with a hand blender, adding more stock if you like a looser consistency. Season to taste and serve topped with ¼ cup grated cheese (add 160 calories), or a few toasted nuts (add 60 calories).

210 CALORIES

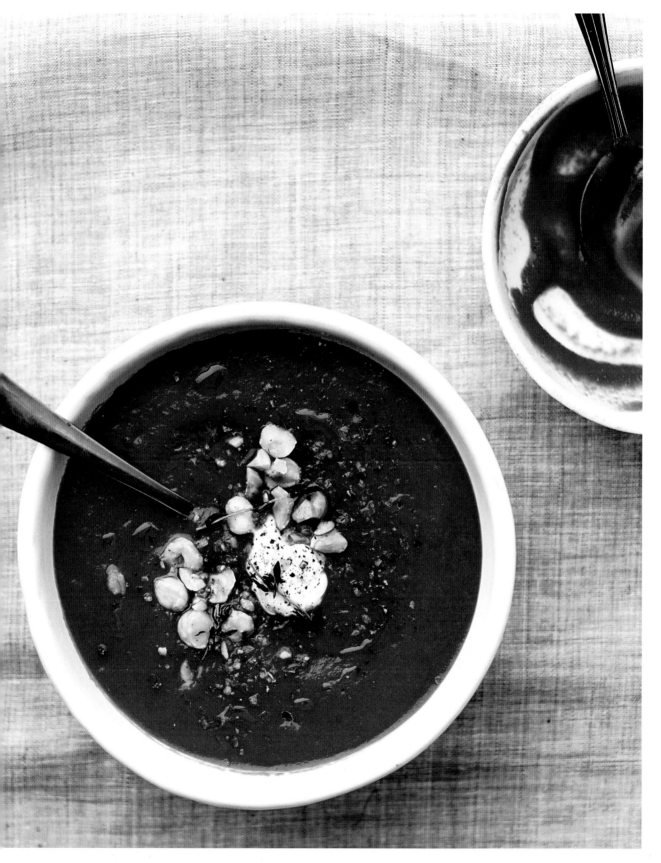

Food to Go, Dips, Spreads, and Crackers

As a GP, I see many patients who have a strong link between gut problems, being overweight or having type 2 diabetes, and busy working lifestyles. It is not easy to find healthy snacks when on the move, and people find themselves grabbing whatever's quickest—often processed, sweet, or starchy food. I hope some of these easy and practical suggestions might help you to break this cycle. Prepare them in advance to save you time in the morning. They will make you feel full for longer, and your microbiome will reward you for it!

Phyto Salad

This salad will provide you with plenty of those all-important anti-inflammatory phytonutrients. While at least three-quarters of your bowl should be plant-based, you should also ensure you get the required fats and proteins. We suggest you choose something from each group below.

3-4 portions of colored vegetables (one can be substituted with fruit), such as:
1 sliced carrot
½ sliced bell pepper (red, orange, yellow)
½ sliced zucchini
5 cherry tomatoes
4 steamed asparagus spears
3-4 artichoke or palm hearts
½ cup radishes, sugar snap peas, or mushrooms
Fruit (about ½ cup): strawberries, unpeeled pear or apple, papaya, mango, grapes,
   pomegranate, blueberries, or raspberries

1-2 cups of greens, such as:
Spinach, mesclun, arugula, kale, broccoli, chicory, cauliflower, bok choy, sprouts,
   Swiss chard, cabbage

1-2 portions of protein, such as:

2 hard-boiled eggs

Meat (about 3 oz): chicken, turkey, cold meat

Fatty fish (about 4 oz): tuna, salmon, mackerel, sardines; or white fish, such as trout, cod, haddock

Dairy (1-2 oz): hard cheese, halloumi, goat cheese, feta

Plant protein: a generous handful of lentils, beans (reduce both of these if you suffer from IBS or bloating), nuts, seeds, tofu, tempeh, hummus

2-3 portions of health-boosting fats, such as:

½ small avocado

6 olives

1-2 tbsp dressing made with extra-virgin olive oil, sesame, walnut, or rapeseed oil

Toasted seeds or nuts: pumpkin seeds, sunflower seeds, pine nuts, hazelnuts, cashews

1-2 portions of beans, squash, or whole grains, such as:

¼ cup cooked quinoa, brown rice, whole barley, or wild red rice

1 slice whole grain bread: millet, spelt, or rye (or gluten-free as required)

¼ cup cooked beans, lentils, or chickpeas

½ cup diced pumpkin or butternut squash

And for extra flavor:

Fermented vegetables, such as sauerkraut or kimchi

Pickled vegetables, such as cornichons, jalapeño peppers, olives

Seaweed: nori cut into strips, kelp/dulse flakes

Fresh herbs: cilantro, mint, parsley, basil, etc.

PHYTONUTRIENTS, also known as phytochemicals, are concentrated in the skins of fruits and vegetables and are responsible for their color, scent, and flavor. The best-known phytonutrients are carotenoids and flavonoids (found in yellow, orange, red, blue, and purple fruits and vegetables), and polyphenols (found in foods like cocoa, olives, tea, coffee, and red wine).

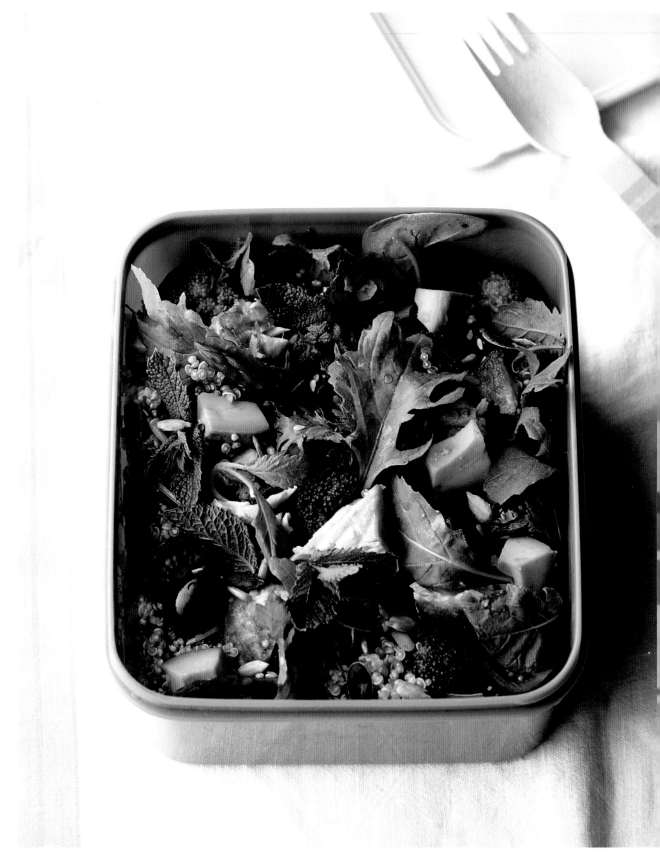

Phyto Salad Lunchbox with Salmon and Avocado

Serves 1

1. Colors

4 asparagus spears,
   steamed and sliced

½ red bell pepper, seeded
   and sliced

5 cherry tomatoes, halved

2. Greens

Small handful of mixed
   greens

4-5 broccoli florets,
   steamed

3. Health-boosting fats

½ avocado, sliced

6 olives

**4. Optional whole grains
   or squash**

¼ cup cooked red and white
   quinoa

5. Proteins

4 oz salmon fillet, grilled

2 tbsp mixed seeds, toasted

And for extra flavor

Handful of fresh mint,
   chopped

Maldon sea salt and
   black pepper

Kefir Mustard Dressing
   (page 119)

•DAIRY-FREE OPTION

•GLUTEN-FREE OPTION

•GOOD FOR PHASE 1

1. In a large bowl, or a plastic container if you're taking it to work, toss together the sliced asparagus, bell pepper, tomatoes, mixed greens, broccoli, avocado, olives, and quinoa.

2. Next add the salmon, and scatter the seeds and mint on top.

3. Make the dressing and put it in a small screw-top jar (if you're taking it to work).

4. When you're ready to eat, season the salad with salt and pepper, pour over the dressing, and toss everything together.

730 CALORIES

Chinese Noodle Jar

Posh pot noodles to take to work—all you need is a spoon and some boiling water. In this recipe you can substitute shrimp or diced chicken for the tofu and add different crunchy vegetables.

Serves 1

Scant 2 oz whole grain soba
  noodles, cooked and
  cooled
5 oz chopped vegetables
  (such as broccoli, bok choy,
  spring greens, sugar snaps,
  mushrooms, bean sprouts)
½ cup shelled edamame
1 small spring onion,
  trimmed and sliced
¼ cup cashews
3 oz firm tofu, cubed
Small handful of fresh
  cilantro, chopped

For the sauce:
2 tsp tamari sauce
1 tsp miso, or ½ vegetable
  bouillon cube
¼ inch fresh ginger, grated
¼ tsp diced red chile
½ tsp sesame oil
2 tsp rice vinegar or raw
  unfiltered apple cider
  vinegar

You will also need:
16-oz jar with screw-top lid
1 small plastic container
  with a tight-fitting lid, for
  the sauce

•DAIRY-FREE
•GLUTEN-FREE
•GOOD FOR PHASE 1

1. Place the noodles, vegetables, edamame, onion, cashews, tofu, and cilantro in the jar in layers so that it is about three-quarters full, and put on the lid.

2. Mix the sauce ingredients in a small plastic container and put on the lid.

3. When you are ready to eat, add ¼ cup hot water to the sauce to loosen it and pour it into the jar, along with an additional ¾-1 cup boiling water. Push the vegetables down into the water and give it all a stir, then allow it to rest for 4-5 minutes. Enjoy directly from the jar or tip it into a bowl.

Tips: Make up extra portions of sauce and keep it in the fridge to use later in the week. You can use other noodles, such as rice noodles, glass noodles (these don't need cooking), or konjac noodles (aka shirataki noodles) which are seriously low-carb.

300 CALORIES

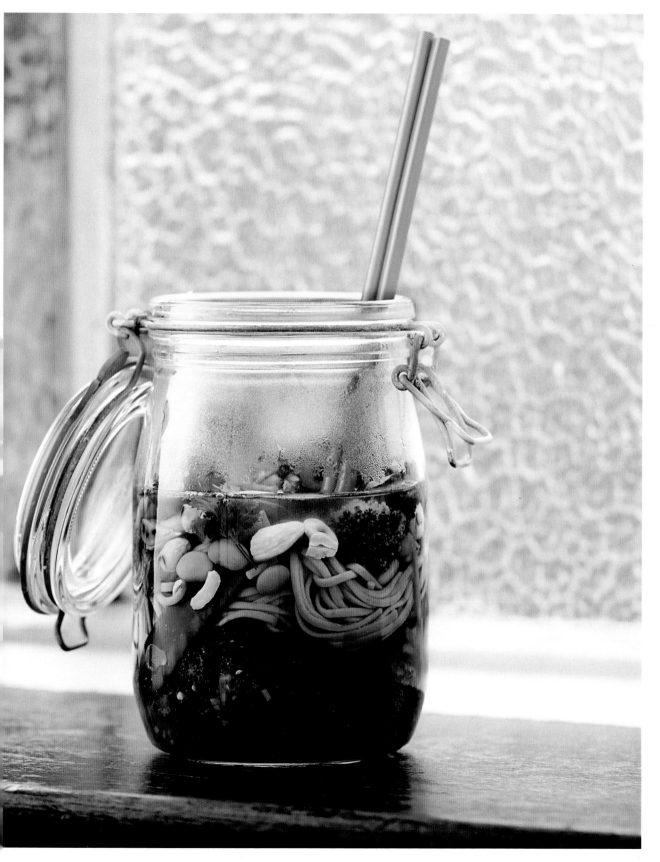

Beet and Yogurt Dip

This vibrant purple dip has a hint of North Africa and is delicious as an accompaniment to a salad or as a colorful side dish.

Serves 4 as a side dish

1 lb beets, scrubbed
   and quartered

¼ cup olive oil

2 large garlic cloves,
   minced

1 tsp ground cumin

½ tsp ground coriander

1 (5-oz) container full-fat
   active Greek-style yogurt
   (or nondairy equivalent)

2 tsp capers, rinsed
   and drained

•DAIRY-FREE OPTION

•GLUTEN-FREE

•GOOD FOR PHASE 1

1. Preheat the oven to 350°F. Toss the beets with the oil, garlic, cumin, and coriander in a roasting pan and roast until tender, 40-50 minutes.

2. Allow them to cool slightly, then blend them in a food processor with the yogurt and capers until they are well combined but still have a bit of texture.

3. Season the dip with sea salt and black pepper. Serve with vegetable crudités, Flaxseed Crackers (page 78), or Whole Grain Flatbread (page 195).

200 CALORIES

Grilled Red Pepper Dip

Chickpeas can moderate your glucose metabolism, and contain resistant starches which produce short-chain fatty acids important for colon health. Even IBS sufferers can usually tolerate them. Instead of grilling red peppers, you could use ½ of a 7-oz jar roasted peppers, drained.

Serves 6 as a dip
(2-4 as a side dish)

2 medium red bell peppers,
  halved and seeded

1 (15-oz) can chickpeas,
  rinsed and drained

5 tbsp extra-virgin olive oil,
  plus more for drizzling

1 tsp salt

1 garlic clove, crushed

Grated zest and juice
  of ½ lemon

Handful of fresh cilantro,
  chopped

½ tsp red pepper flakes,
  or to taste

Large pinch of paprika,
  for serving

• DAIRY-FREE

• GLUTEN-FREE

• GOOD FOR PHASE 1

1. Place the bell pepper halves under a hot broiler, skin side up, or over a flame until the skin has charred. Put them in a resealable bag to let them sweat, which helps to loosen the skin. Once they have cooled, remove the skin and place them in a food processor with the remaining ingredients.

2. Blitz until you have a smooth paste.

3. Serve the dip drizzled with a little oil and a sprinkling of paprika and some vegetable crudités on the side.

Tip: You can substitute the chickpeas with butter beans, though these can exacerbate IBS symptoms in some people so are probably best avoided and only added in Phase 2. Like chickpeas, they are rich in protein, fiber, iron, and B vitamins.

160 CALORIES

Lemon-Cilantro Hummus with Seaweed

Tahini paste is made from ground sesame seeds, and when combined with chickpeas provides an ideal balance of amino acids for protein absorption. The seaweed adds lovely marine omega-3s.

Serves 6

1 (15-oz) can chickpeas, drained and rinsed

1 large garlic clove, peeled

1 tbsp tahini

2 tbsp full-fat active Greek-style yogurt (or nondairy equivalent)

1 tbsp Preserved Lemons (page 184), seeds removed (or zest and juice of 1 lemon)

3 tbsp olive oil, plus more for drizzling

1 nori seaweed sheet, finely sliced, plus a little extra for garnish

Large handful of fresh cilantro, including stalks, chopped

•DAIRY-FREE OPTION

•GLUTEN-FREE

•GOOD FOR PHASE 1

1. Blitz all the ingredients except the cilantro in a food processor, leaving a bit of texture. Add the cilantro and pulse briefly.

2. Leave it to rest for 30 minutes to bring out the flavors (if time permits). Drizzle with oil and garnish with a few slices of chopped seaweed before serving.

140 CALORIES

Avocado and Lime Salsa

Creamy, tangy, and slightly piquant, this makes a marvelous dip or accompaniment to a meal. It is full of nutrients and natural fats.

Serves 2
1 avocado, diced
½ red onion, finely diced
½-1 tsp red pepper flakes
  to taste
1 tbsp chopped fresh
  cilantro or basil
1 tbsp lime juice
½ tbsp olive oil, for drizzling

•DAIRY-FREE
•GLUTEN-FREE
•GOOD FOR PHASE 1

1. Place all the ingredients except the oil in a dish and mash them together. Season with Maldon sea salt and freshly ground black pepper and drizzle with the oil.

2. Serve the salsa as a dip with vegetable crudités, or as a side dish with fish.

Smoked Mackerel Pâté

Mouthwatering, quick to make, and full of essential omega-3 fats.

Serves 4
5 oz smoked mackerel
  fillets, skinned
3 tbsp full-fat active Greek-
  style yogurt (or nondairy
  equivalent)
½ tsp prepared horseradish
Juice of 1 lemon

•DAIRY-FREE OPTION
•GLUTEN-FREE
•GOOD FOR PHASE 1

1. Flake the fish into a dish, add the remaining ingredients, and mix well. Season with freshly ground black pepper.

2. Serve with Flaxseed Crackers (page 78) or Thai-Flavored Seaweed Crackers (page 79), or spread it on Spinach and Ricotta Blinis (page 80).

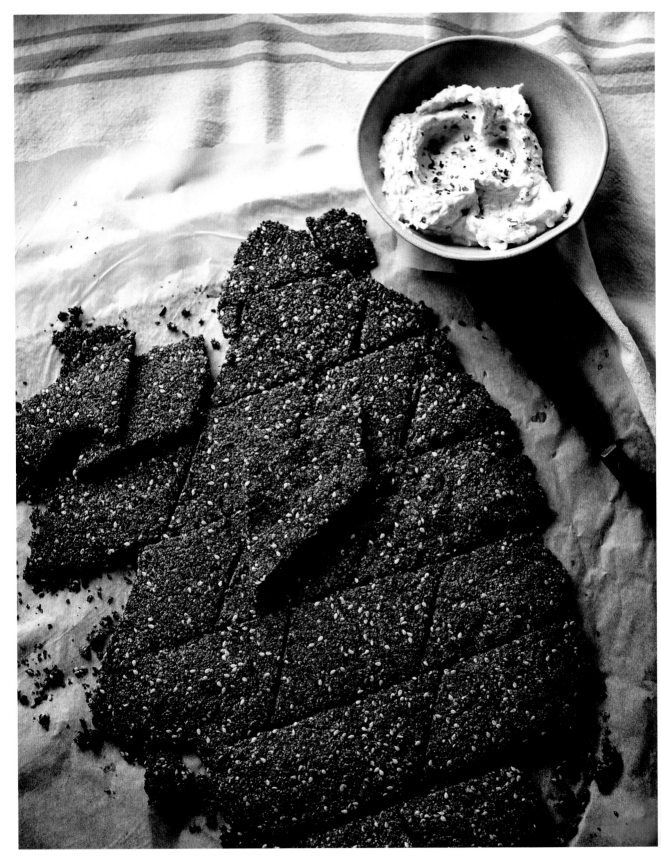

3 Cream Cheese Spreads

Dairy is thankfully no longer seen as one of the major causes of cardiovascular disease and diabetes. In fact, recent research suggests that it may even have a beneficial effect on these conditions. It's also a great source of calcium and protein. These spreads taste great served on rye bread, our Flaxseed Crackers (see page 78; shown left, with the horseradish spread), or simply on thinly sliced, toasted whole wheat soda bread.

Each serves 2

Horseradish Spread

5 oz full-fat cream cheese
2 tsp prepared horseradish
1 tsp rosemary leaves,
    finely chopped

Mix the ingredients in a bowl and serve as a dip or spread.

Smoked Salmon Spread

5 oz full-fat cream cheese
2 oz smoked salmon, diced
Juice of ½ lemon
Small handful of fresh dill,
    chopped
Black pepper

Mix the ingredients in a bowl and serve as a dip or spread.

Beet and Chile Spread

5 oz full-fat cream cheese
⅔ cup diced cooked beets
2 tsp chopped chives
1 tsp lemon juice
Pinch of red pepper flakes

•ALL GLUTEN-FREE

Blend the cream cheese with half the beets, the chives, lemon juice, and red pepper flakes in a small food processor until smooth. Stir in the remaining beets and season with black pepper.

Flaxseed Crackers

Flaxseed is fast becoming another popular super food, packed as it is with protein, omega-3s, vitamins, and minerals. These crackers also contain lignans, which have strong antioxidant properties and may help prevent some common cancers.

Makes about 20 crackers
200g (1¾ cups) ground flaxseeds
50g (½ cup) sesame seeds
2 tbsp chia seeds
1 tsp yeast extract (or
   1 tbsp vegan yeast if
   you're gluten-sensitive)
½ tsp Maldon sea salt

•DAIRY-FREE
•GLUTEN-FREE OPTION
•GOOD FOR PHASE 1

1. Preheat the oven to 250°F. Place the flaxseeds, sesame seeds, and chia seeds in a bowl.

2. Dissolve the yeast in a scant ¼ cup boiling water, then add a scant ½ cup cold water. Pour it into the seed mixture and stir vigorously until you have a gloopy paste. If it is dry or crumbly, add a little more water. Leave it to firm up for about 10 minutes.

3. Spread the mixture on parchment paper or a silicone baking sheet. Place another piece of parchment paper on top and use a rolling pin to flatten it to approximately ⅛-inch thickness. Remove the top piece of parchment paper and lightly score the surface so the dough can be separated into 20 square crackers. Scatter the salt over it.

4. Bake the dough in the middle of the oven for 30-40 minutes, until it is just starting to turn golden brown around the edges. Check it frequently, as it will taste bitter if you overcook it. Turn it over, then turn off the oven and leave it to dry out for at least 30 minutes. Once it has cooled, break it up into squares. The crackers will keep for up to 5 days in an airtight container.

Tip: If using vegan yeast, add it to the bowl with the seeds before adding the water.

80 CALORIES PER CRACKER

Thai-Flavored Seaweed Crackers

These irresistible gluten-free crackers are high in fiber and give a good seaweed boost. You and your biome will love them. Try them with a dip, crumbled into a soup, or simply savor them on their own.

Makes about 24 crackers

100g (¾ cup) buckwheat flour

100g (scant 1 cup) ground flaxseeds

50g (½ cup) sesame seeds

2 nori seaweed sheets, chopped

½ tsp red pepper flakes (optional)

1 tbsp Thai fish sauce

2 tbsp tamari sauce

1 tsp sesame oil

•DAIRY-FREE

•GLUTEN-FREE

•GOOD FOR PHASE 1

1. Preheat the oven to 250°F. Place the flour, flaxseeds, sesame seeds, nori, and red pepper flakes, if using, in a bowl.

2. Add 3-4 tbsp water along with the Thai fish sauce and tamari sauce and stir vigorously to produce a very wet, sticky dough. If it is dry or crumbly, add more water gradually. Leave it to rest and firm up for about 10 minutes.

3. Spread the mixture on parchment paper or a silicone baking sheet lightly greased with sesame oil. Place another greased piece of parchment paper on top and use a rolling pin to roll it to a ⅛-inch thickness. Remove the top piece of parchment and lightly score the surface so the dough can be separated into 24 square crackers.

4. Bake the dough in the middle of the oven for 30-40 minutes, until it is just starting to turn golden brown around the edges. Check it frequently, as it will taste bitter if overcooked. Turn it over, then turn off the oven and leave it to dry out for at least 30 minutes. Let it cool completely on a wire rack before breaking it up into squares. The crackers will keep for up to 5 days in an airtight container.

160 CALORIES PER CRACKER

Spinach and Ricotta Blinis

Delicious green blinis that are packed with nutrients and work brilliantly with our spreads (page 77) and dips (pages 72-73). They can be included in Phase 1, as cheese tends to be better tolerated than milk and the quantity in each blini is small, but best avoid them if you are dairy-intolerant.

Makes 8-10

5 oz fresh spinach
(or thawed frozen
and drained)
½ cup whole wheat
buckwheat flour
1 tsp baking powder
¼ cup grated Parmesan
2 eggs
Scant ½ cup ricotta
2-3 tbsp milk (or nondairy
equivalent)
2 tbsp olive oil

• GLUTEN-FREE
• GOOD FOR PHASE 1

1. Place the spinach in a colander and pour over boiling water, then refresh it under a cold running tap. Drain it well and squeeze out as much water as possible before chopping finely.

2. Mix the flour, baking powder, and Parmesan in a bowl with salt and pepper.

3. Beat the eggs with the ricotta and pour them into the flour mixture, whisking in enough milk to produce a thick batter. Stir in the spinach.

4. Heat the oil in a large frying pan. Add the batter to the pan in batches of 3 or 4, using a tablespoon of the batter for each blini. Cook until they are golden brown, 3-4 minutes per side, then place them on paper towels to drain.

Tip: These are delicious topped with smoked salmon, a squeeze of lemon, and some freshly ground black pepper.

120 CALORIES PER BLINI

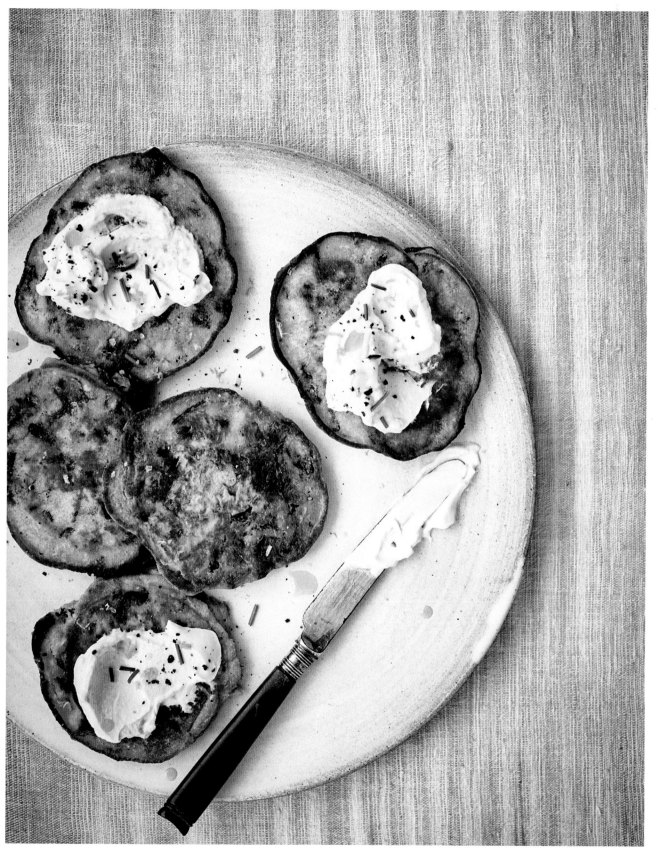

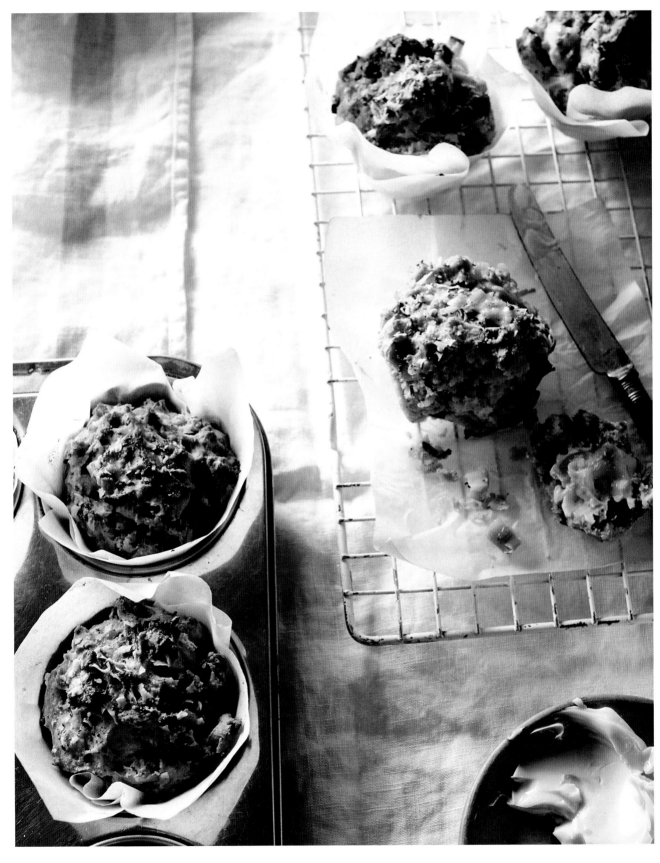

Sour Cream and Seaweed Muffins

Put one of these in your bag as you leave home. A tasty, nutritious snack to keep you from temptation . . .

Makes 12

50g (3½ tbsp) butter

4 spring onions, trimmed
  and finely chopped

2 large eggs

150ml (scant ⅔ cup)
  buttermilk

160g (½ cup) sour cream
  and chive dip

1½ sheets nori seaweed,
  finely chopped

260g (2⅛ cups) whole
  grain flour, such as
  buckwheat or spelt

¼ cup grated Parmesan

1 tsp baking powder

•GLUTEN-FREE
•GOOD FOR PHASE 1

1. Preheat the oven to 350°F. Line a 12-well muffin pan with paper liners.

2. Melt the butter in a small frying pan and cook the onions for 3-4 minutes. In a bowl, beat together the eggs, buttermilk, and sour cream dip, then stir in the cooked onions and the seaweed.

3. In a separate bowl, mix the flour, Parmesan, and baking powder and season with salt and plenty of freshly ground black pepper. Make a well in the center of the dry ingredients and pour in the egg mixture. Combine everything well, but take care not to overmix.

4. Spoon the mixture into the muffin cups and bake for 18-20 minutes, or until the tops are golden. They taste good hot or cold.

Tip: These muffins freeze well.

200 CALORIES EACH

Smoked Salmon Ceviche

This mildly exotic-tasting fatty fish salad is ideal for a fasting-day lunch. Smoked salmon is remarkably filling yet low in calories. You also get some added protein, nutrients, and fiber from the edamame.

Serves 1

Juice of 1 lime, or ½-1 tbsp yuzu juice

1 tbsp raw unfiltered organic apple cider vinegar

½ tsp mirin wine, or ¼ tsp sugar

¼ tsp finely grated fresh ginger

Pinch of cayenne pepper or mild chili powder

2 oz smoked salmon, diced

⅓ cup cooked shelled edamame

2-3 radishes, thinly sliced

1 cup watercress

½ avocado, diced

1 tbsp mild olive oil

•DAIRY-FREE

•GLUTEN-FREE

•GOOD FOR PHASE 1

1. Mix the lime juice, vinegar, mirin, ginger, and cayenne in a bowl. Stir in the salmon, edamame, and radishes and let the mixture marinate for 30 minutes.

2. When you are ready to eat, toss the watercress and avocado in the oil in another bowl and place the salmon mixture on top.

Tips: Diced off-cuts of smoked salmon work fine and are far cheaper. Alternatively use 5 oz good-quality fillet of salmon cut into small cubes. Yuzu is a Japanese citrus fruit with a particularly tangy and sharp flavor—it is available in some supermarkets.

450 CALORIES

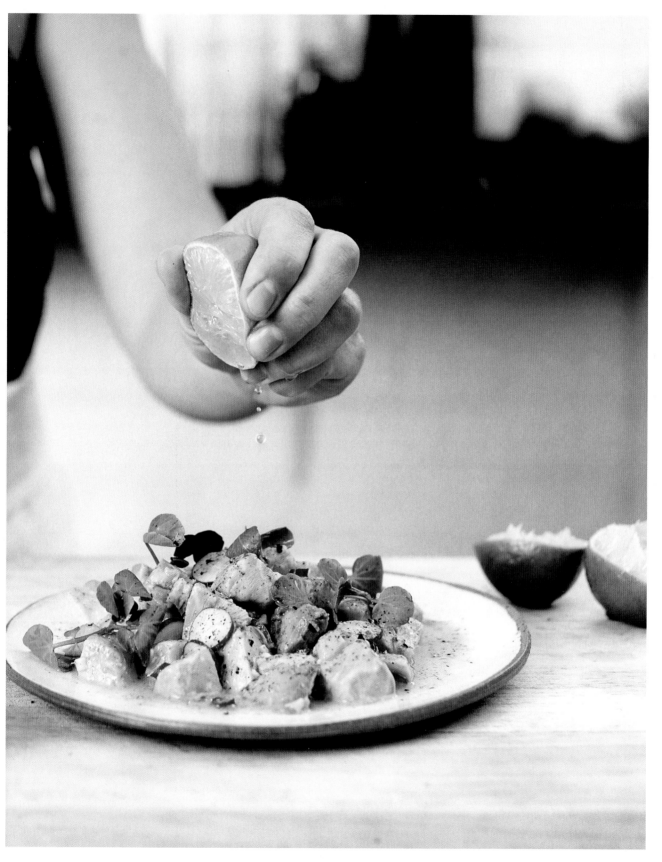

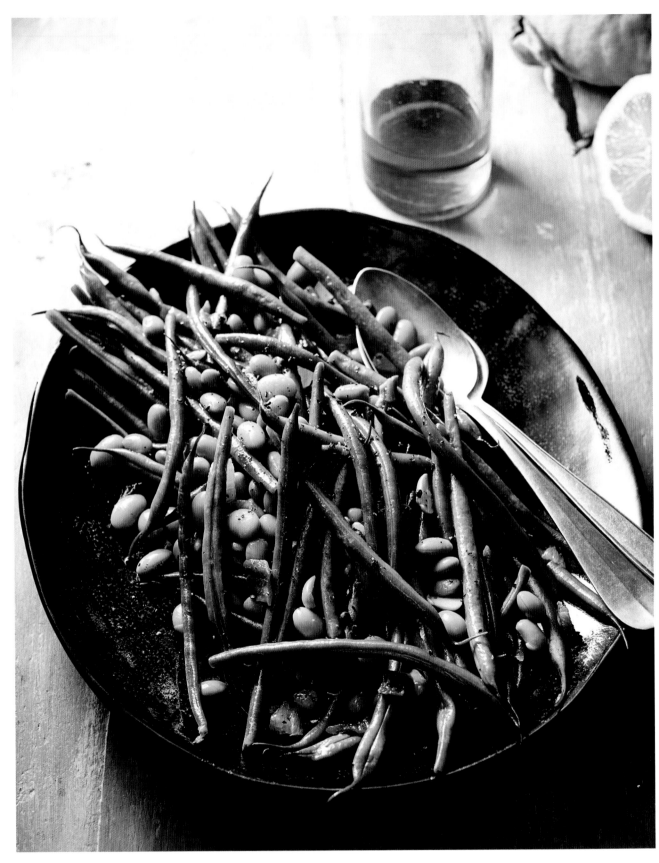

Green Beans and Edamame with Anchovies

This salad contains a good amount of protein and plenty of fiber to nourish your microbiome.

Serves 2

8 salt-packed anchovies, rinsed and chopped

Juice of ½ lemon

2 tbsp olive oil

¾ cup frozen shelled edamame

5 oz thin green beans, trimmed

•DAIRY-FREE

•GLUTEN-FREE

1. Mix the anchovies with the lemon juice and oil in a medium bowl.

2. Bring a pan of salted water to a boil and add the edamame. Bring it back to a boil and add the green beans. Cook for 3-4 minutes, until the beans are al dente. Drain, then stir them into the anchovy mixture. Add a generous grinding of black pepper and serve.

Note: In Phase 1 you may wish to reduce your portion size as the "scratchy" fibers in both beans can exacerbate IBS.

240 CALORIES

Warm Lentil Salad

Serves 2

¾ cup Puy lentils, rinsed

1 garlic clove

1 bay leaf

1 red onion, finely chopped

3 medium tomatoes, chopped

1⅔ cups spinach

1 tbsp balsamic vinegar

2 tbsp extra-virgin olive oil

½ cup chopped firm goat cheese (or nondairy cheese)

Handful of fresh parsley, chopped

•DAIRY-FREE OPTION

•GLUTEN-FREE

1. Place the lentils in a saucepan with the garlic, bay leaf, and 2 cups of cold water. Bring to a boil, reduce the heat, and simmer for 20 minutes, or until the lentils are tender.

2. Drain the lentils, discarding the garlic and bay leaf, and leave them to cool for 5 minutes in a salad bowl.

3. Stir the remaining ingredients into the warm lentils, season well with salt and freshly ground black pepper, and sprinkle with parsley to serve.

Note: Lentils can make IBS worse. Reduce or avoid in Phase 1.

440 CALORIES

Terra Mare Salad

This salad is so nutritious it's hard to know where to start. In fact, it may be the most gut-friendly recipe in this book . . . It has diverse dietary fiber from both sea and land, as well as other important metabolites linked to gut health. It was given to us by marine conservationist and sustainable seaweed producer, Dr. Pia Winberg.

Serves 2

½ cup quinoa
4 tbsp olive oil
2 leeks, diced
8 oz squid (fresh or frozen)
2 tbsp dukkah
¼ oz nori seaweed sheets,
   finely chopped
1 lemon, ½ for juice and
   ½ cut into wedges
Arugula and baby
   spinach leaves

•DAIRY-FREE
•GLUTEN-FREE
•GOOD FOR PHASE 1

1. Rinse the quinoa well and cook it according to the package instructions.

2. Heat 2 tbsp of the oil in a frying pan and sauté the leek gently for 6-8 minutes.

3. Meanwhile, cut open the squid, lay it flat with the inside facing up and crisscross the surface with a sharp knife. Slice it into ½-inch strips.

4. In another frying pan, heat the remaining 2 tbsp oil and stir-fry the squid for a couple of minutes, taking care not to overcook it or it will be rubbery.

5. Blend the dukkah spice with the nori. Remove the squid from the heat and toss it in the dukkah mix, the lemon juice and some salt and pepper. Mix it in a large bowl with the quinoa, leeks, arugula, and baby spinach. Serve with the lemon wedges.

400 CALORIES

SEAWEEDS have uniquely high levels of soluble dietary fiber (over 25 percent of their dry weight) and provide one of the best sources of the anti-inflammatory omega-3 fatty acids. Studies have shown that seaweed increases specific beneficial bacteria in the gut that are known to protect the mucous lining, as well as reduce inflammation.

Toasted Slaw with Halloumi and Lemony Buttermilk Dressing

The broccoli and red cabbage in this dish boost your phytonutrient intake and the buttermilk dressing boosts your probiotics. By heating and slightly toasting the crisper vegetables you make them easier to digest.

Serves 2

1½ cups thinly sliced red cabbage leaves

1½ cups thinly sliced green cabbage leaves

4 oz broccoli, cut into bite-size pieces

2 tbsp olive oil

2 oz shiitake or cremini mushrooms, sliced

5 oz halloumi, sliced

Generous handful of bitter greens (spinach, arugula, or dandelion greens)

½ recipe Lemony Buttermilk Dressing (page 118)

1 tbsp slivered almonds, toasted

•GLUTEN-FREE

1. Scorch the cabbage and broccoli on a very hot grill pan, turning them once. This should take about 2 minutes on each side. Then tip them into a wide salad bowl.

2. Heat the oil in a frying pan and fry the mushrooms and halloumi slices until they are golden. Stir them into the cabbage mixture.

3. Add the greens and toss everything with the Lemony Buttermilk Dressing. Sprinkle the almonds on top before serving.

530 CALORIES WITH DRESSING

Warm Red Rice Salad with Zucchini

Serves 2

⅔ cup cooked red
  Camargue rice
2 zucchini, sliced
¼ small cabbage, sliced
⅓ cup pine nuts, toasted
1 tbsp diced Preserved
  Lemons (page 184)
Juice of 1 lemon
2 tbsp extra-virgin olive oil
2 tbsp chopped fresh
  parsley
1 tsp chopped fresh mint
2 tsp chopped fresh thyme

•DAIRY-FREE
•GLUTEN-FREE
•GOOD FOR PHASE 1

1. Reheat the rice by adding 1 tbsp water and zapping it in a microwave or steaming it in a pan. Spoon into a salad bowl.

2. Place the zucchini slices and cabbage on a very hot grill pan for a couple of minutes, turning them as they char. Stir them into the rice, along with the rest of the ingredients.

Tip: If you don't have preserved lemons, you can use the grated zest of 1 lemon.

Broccoli and Asparagus with Buttermilk Dressing

Serves 2

¼ head broccoli
¼ cauliflower
1 small bunch asparagus,
  tips only
2 tbsp pumpkin seeds
1 head romaine lettuce,
  sliced
¼ red onion, thinly sliced
½ recipe Turmeric
  Buttermilk Dressing
  (page 119)
⅔ cup crumbled feta

•GLUTEN-FREE

1. Break the broccoli and cauliflower into florets and place them in a hot grill pan for 3-4 minutes, turning them as they char. Tip them into a serving bowl, then cook the asparagus in the same way and add to the bowl.

2. Toast the pumpkin seeds in a small pan until they start to pop, then remove from the heat. Once the vegetables have cooled a bit, add the lettuce and onion and toss everything with the dressing. Scatter the feta and pumpkin seeds on top.

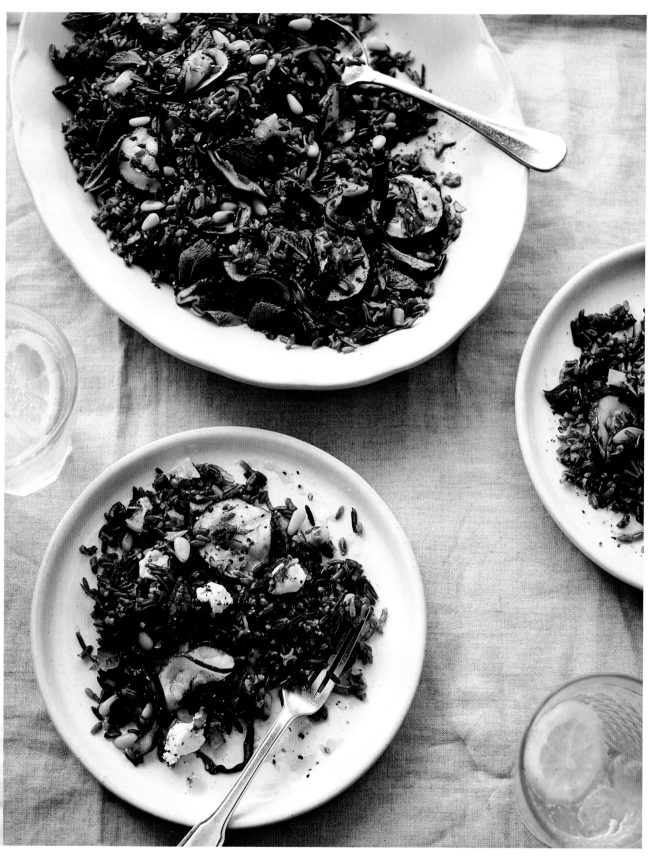

Low-Carb Mac 'n' Cheese

Macaroni and cheese is experiencing a renaissance, a classic home-cooked comfort food that is now being served in top restaurants. Here is a relatively low-carb version that is creamy, nutritious, and satisfying, with a mild chile kick.

Serves 2

3 oz green-pea macaroni
   (or other gluten-free
   whole grain macaroni)
1 cup cauliflower florets
1 cup broccoli florets
2 tbsp olive oil
1 garlic clove, crushed
½-1 green jalapeño chile
   from a jar, diced
¾ cup grated aged Cheddar
   cheese
⅔ cup crème fraîche
¼ cup grated Parmesan

•GLUTEN-FREE

1. Preheat the oven to 350°F. Cook the pasta according to the package instructions until al dente. Drain and rinse under cold running water.

2. Toss the cauliflower and broccoli florets in the oil and a generous pinch of salt, then spread out on a baking sheet or in a roasting pan. Bake for 10-15 minutes or until they start to brown around the edges, then transfer them to a medium baking dish. Stir in the pasta with the garlic and chile.

3. In a bowl, mix together the Cheddar and crème fraîche. Spread this mixture on top of the vegetables, followed by a sprinkling of Parmesan and freshly ground black pepper.

4. Bake for 12-15 minutes or until the top is turning golden brown and the cheesy sauce is bubbling.

Tip: This is delicious served with Green Beans and Edamame with Anchovies (page 87).

750 CALORIES

Kale and Tofu Scramble

A spicy vegan alternative to scrambled eggs. Very tasty as well.

Serves 2

3 tbsp olive oil

1 tsp cumin seeds

½ tsp paprika

8 oz firm tofu, chopped
   into ¾-inch pieces

4 cups cauliflower florets

½ cup pine nuts

2 large handfuls kale,
   chopped, tough stalks
   removed

2 tbsp fresh cilantro,
   chopped

•DAIRY-FREE
•GLUTEN-FREE
•GOOD FOR PHASE 1

1. Preheat the oven to 350°F. In a bowl, mix together the oil, spices, salt, and pepper. Stir in the tofu, followed by the cauliflower.

2. Spread the mixture in a roasting pan and bake for 20 minutes, stirring from time to time until slightly brown. Scatter the pine nuts on top 5 minutes before the end of the cooking time.

3. Meanwhile, steam the kale until just tender, 2-3 minutes, then divide it between 2 plates. Scatter the cauliflower and tofu mixture over the top, and finish with a sprinkling of cilantro.

Tip: Instead of steaming the kale you can stir it into the roasting pan with the tofu and cauliflower when you add the pine nuts.

580 CALORIES

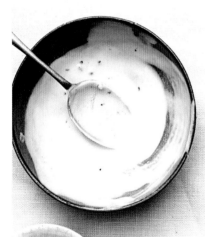

Mustard seeds enhance the absorption of glucosinolates (which are thought to protect against inflammation and some cancers) from cruciferous vegetables such as cauliflower, cabbage, kale, Brussels sprouts, and broccoli.

Cauliflower Baked with Lemon and Almonds

A scrumptious alternative to starchy potatoes, and one that your gut bacteria will love.

Serves 4

1 large cauliflower, cut into florets

¼ cup extra-virgin olive oil

1 tbsp Preserved Lemons (page 184), or grated zest and juice of 1 lemon

½ tsp red pepper flakes

1 tsp mustard seeds

½ cup slivered almonds

Juice of 1 lemon

•DAIRY-FREE

•GLUTEN-FREE

•GOOD FOR PHASE 1

1. Preheat the oven to 350°F. Spread the florets in a large roasting pan.

2. Drizzle over the oil and season well with sea salt and freshly ground black pepper. Bake for 10 minutes.

3. Remove from the oven, mix in the preserved lemons and red pepper flakes, and scatter over the mustard seeds and almonds. Bake for another 10-12 minutes, or until the cauliflower is tender and browning in places. Transfer to a serving dish and drizzle over the lemon juice before serving.

Tip: For added flavor you can whip up a tahini drizzle, with 2 tbsp tahini, 1 tbsp fresh lemon juice, and 1 tbsp warm water, seasoned with salt and pepper (add 60 calories). And for a bit more crunch and color you might scatter on some pomegranate seeds a few minutes before serving. (Avoid pomegranate during Phase 1 as its tough fiber can exacerbate IBS symptoms.)

220 CALORIES

Eggplant Parmigiana

A delicious, Mediterranean-style bake. Eggplant contains antioxidants such as anthocyanin, a pigment that, among other things, can protect against cellular damage.

Serves 2

1 large eggplant, cut into
 ½-inch slices
4 tbsp olive oil
1 garlic clove, minced
2 tsp fresh oregano,
 chopped (or 1 tsp dried)
⅔ cup passata (or strained
 crushed tomatoes)
4 oz mozzarella (or nondairy
 cheese), sliced
Handful of cherry tomatoes,
 halved
½ cup grated Parmesan
 (or vegan Parmesan)

•DAIRY-FREE OPTION
•GLUTEN-FREE
•GOOD FOR PHASE 1

1. Preheat the oven to 350°F. Brush the eggplant slices on both sides with 3 tbsp of the oil, then brown them on a very hot grill pan.

2. Stir the garlic and oregano into the passata and pour it into a baking dish. Lay the eggplant slices on top, followed by the mozzarella and the cherry tomatoes. Drizzle over the remaining 1 tbsp oil, and finish with a sprinkling of Parmesan.

3. Bake the parmigiana for 14-15 minutes, or until the top is lightly golden. Serve with a crisp green salad.

Tip: Throw in a handful of pitted olives for extra flavor (add 20 calories).

580 CALORIES

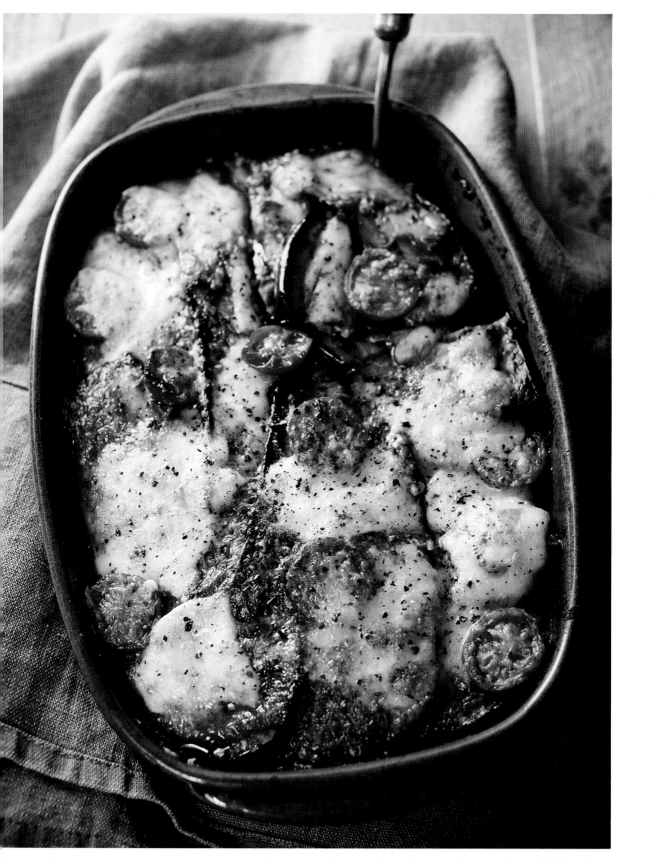

Michael's Mussels

A firm favorite in our household, and one that brings out the hunter-gatherer in Michael, who relishes scrubbing and preparing the mussels. Having said that, mussels are usually so well cleaned these days that there is hardly a tuft of seaweed beard left on them to remove. Mussels are probably the most sustainable source of high-quality protein you will find. Fussy to eat, but worth it—savor their delicate, sweet, and juicy flesh.

Serves 2

2¼ lb fresh mussels in shells

2 tbsp olive oil

½ onion, finely diced

1 garlic clove, crushed
   or minced

½ cup white wine

Sprig of fresh thyme

2 tbsp crème fraîche
   (optional)

Generous handful of fresh
   parsley, chopped

•DAIRY-FREE OPTION

•GLUTEN-FREE

•GOOD FOR PHASE 1

1. Check each mussel shell to make sure it closes when you tap it. Discard any that remain open when tapped—the mussels need to be fresh and alive. Scrub off any obvious chunks of seaweed.

2. Heat the oil in a Dutch oven over medium heat and sauté the onion for about 5 minutes, adding the garlic after 3 minutes.

3. Pour in the wine, followed by the thyme and mussels. Cover the pan with a well-fitting lid and bring it to a boil. Cook for 4-5 minutes or until the mussels have opened. Discard any that remain shut.

4. Divide the mussels between 2 bowls, reserving the juices. Stir the crème fraîche (if using) and parsley into the juices before pouring them over the mussels. Serve them with chunks of fresh No-Knead Sourdough (page 198) or Whole Grain Flatbread (page 195) and a bitter greens salad.

370 CALORIES

Pasta with Pistachio Pesto

Made with pistachio nuts, this rich creamy pesto has a gorgeous subtle flavor. You'll never want to go back to a store-bought jar. Mixing spaghetti with some spiralized zucchini is a great pain-free way of reducing your carb consumption.

Serves 4

Pistachio Pesto

4 cups fresh basil leaves
¾ cup grated Parmesan
  (or vegan Parmesan)
1 cup pistachios
2 garlic cloves, chopped
⅔ cup olive oil

Pasta

6 oz whole wheat spaghetti
  (or gluten-free
  alternative)
4 medium zucchini or
  10 oz butternut squash,
  spiralized

•DAIRY-FREE OPTION
•GLUTEN-FREE OPTION
•GOOD FOR PHASE 1

1. To make the pesto, blend the basil, Parmesan, pistachios, and garlic in a food processor until they start to break down. Gradually add the oil until the mixture starts to thicken into a sauce. Season to taste with salt and pepper.

2. Cook the spaghetti in salted water according to the package instructions. Add the zucchini for the last minute of cooking. Drain the pasta and vegetables and tip them into a large serving bowl. Stir in the pesto so everything gets a good coating. Serve immediately.

Tip: If you buy 3 pots of basil from the supermarket or farmers' market and pinch off the large and medium leaves, leaving the small ones to grow, you will be able to make the pesto again in a few weeks' time.

580 CALORIES

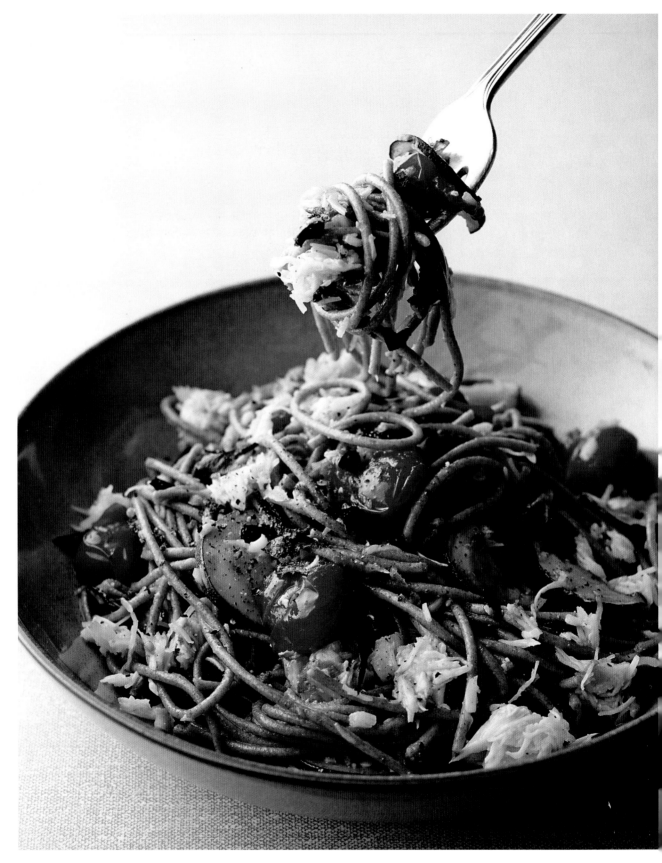

Crab Spaghetti with Seaweed

Crab is a great source of protein and selenium, which has anti-inflammatory properties. Its slightly sweet taste is enhanced here by the umami flavors of seaweed.

Serves 2

8-10 oz whole grain spaghetti or green-pea pasta (or gluten-free alternative)

3 tbsp olive oil

2-3 garlic cloves, finely chopped

1 red chile, seeded and finely chopped, or ½ tsp red pepper flakes

10 grape or cherry tomatoes

1 zucchini, halved lengthwise and sliced

8 oz crab meat (fresh, canned, or frozen)

Juice of ½ large lemon

Large handful of fresh parsley, coarsely chopped

1 nori seaweed sheet, chopped

•DAIRY-FREE
•GLUTEN-FREE OPTION
•GOOD FOR PHASE 1

1. Cook the pasta according to the package instructions. Drain it when it is al dente, retaining 2 tbsp of the cooking water, then rinse under cold running water and set aside.

2. Meanwhile, heat the oil in a large frying pan and gently fry the garlic, chile, tomatoes, and zucchini for 2-3 minutes. Stir in the crab meat and heat it through, then add the lemon juice.

3. Add the cooked pasta, along with the reserved cooking water, parsley, and nori. Stir well to warm the pasta through and ensure it gets a good even coating of the sauce. Season and serve with a dark green leaf salad.

800 CALORIES

Poor Man's Potatoes with Anchovies

Based on a classic Spanish dish *papas a lo pobre*, this makes a wonderfully comforting, easy meal.

Serves 4

1 lb baby new potatoes, halved

5 tbsp olive oil

1 large red onion, thinly sliced

1 large green bell pepper, seeded and thinly sliced

2 large garlic cloves, thinly sliced

½ (2-oz) jar anchovies, drained and chopped

Juice of ½ lemon

Sprig of fresh rosemary or thyme

Large handful of fresh parsley, chopped

•DAIRY-FREE

•GLUTEN-FREE

•GOOD FOR PHASE 1

1. Ideally, use precooked potatoes, i.e., ones that have been boiled for 15-20 minutes in lightly salted water until they're tender, then cooled in the fridge for 12 hours to bring out the resistant starch. Otherwise, boil the potatoes and use them immediately.

2. Heat the oil in a large frying pan and sweat the onion and bell pepper for 5 minutes before adding the potatoes.

3. Add the garlic and cook for 1-2 minutes, then stir in the anchovies, lemon juice, and rosemary sprig.

4. Sauté for 5 minutes, stirring occasionally, until the vegetables are tender but not browned. Season generously with black pepper and stir in the parsley. Serve with a multicolored salad or other colorful vegetables.

Note: Anyone with active IBS may need to reduce the amount of onions and garlic.

260 CALORIES

Green peppers are an excellent source of vitamins A, C, and B6. Anchovies provide lots of lovely omega-3s . . .

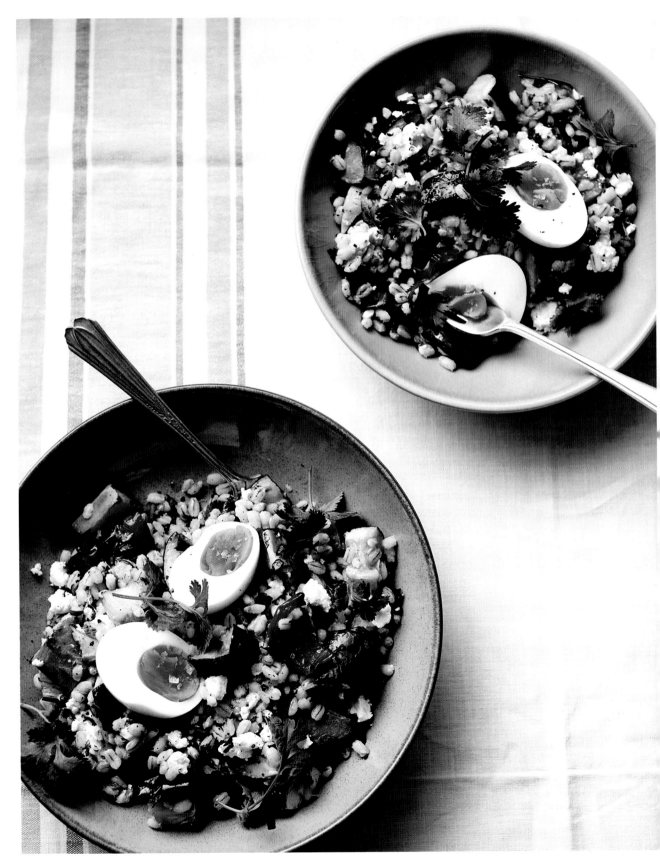

Roasted Mediterranean Vegetables, Pearl Barley, and Eggs

If you haven't tried pearl barley, here's a chance. Slow to release its starches, this delicious whole grain provides a steady source of energy and delivers more fiber to feed your biome than the more processed grains. Serve warm or cold.

Serves 2

1 small eggplant, diced

1 large zucchini, sliced

1 red bell pepper, seeded and sliced

¾ cup cubed butternut squash

3 tbsp olive oil

½ cup pearl barley

2 hard-boiled eggs, quartered

½ cup crumbled goat cheese (or nondairy cheese)

Handful of fresh parsley or cilantro, chopped

Juice of ½ lemon

• DAIRY-FREE OPTION

• GOOD FOR PHASE 1

1. Preheat the oven to 390°F. Place the eggplant, zucchini, bell pepper, and squash in a roasting pan and toss with the oil, salt, and pepper.

2. Bake the vegetables for 30-40 minutes, or until they're tender and browned at the edges, turning them once or twice.

3. Meanwhile, cook the pearl barley according to the package instructions.

4. Remove the vegetables from the oven and stir in the barley. Transfer everything to a serving dish, lightly stir in the eggs, and scatter the goat cheese and parsley on top. Season to taste with Maldon sea salt, black pepper, and lemon juice.

Tip: For a gluten-free version, swap the pearl barley for gluten-free quinoa or buckwheat. This is an ideal recipe for using up leftover grains, which of course contain extra gut-friendly resistant starch if they have been cooled in the fridge before being reheated.

520 CALORIES

Mackerel with Quinoa Tabbouleh

Of all the fatty fish, mackerel has one of the highest concentrations of omega-3s. Quinoa, meanwhile, is truly a miracle grain, containing thiamine, which helps create the digestive acids in your stomach; riboflavin, which is crucial for the health of the gut wall; and also amino acids such as glutamine, a primary source of energy for the gut, helping it produce adequate amounts of protective mucus—something that is particularly important during periods of strenuous exercise, stress, or medical trauma.

Serves 4

1⅓ cups quinoa

¾ cup diced cooked beets

1 carrot, grated

Large handful of fresh parsley, chopped

Large handful of fresh mint, chopped

Large handful of fresh cilantro, chopped

Large handful of chives, chopped

1 tbsp pine nuts, lightly toasted

½ cucumber, diced

Juice of 1 lime

2 tbsp extra-virgin olive oil

4 large mackerel fillets

•DAIRY-FREE

•GLUTEN-FREE

•GOOD FOR PHASE 1

1. Cook the quinoa according to the package instructions, then drain and refresh under cold running water. Put in a large bowl and stir in the beets, carrot, herbs, pine nuts, and cucumber. Add the lime juice, oil, salt, pepper and mix everything together. Let stand at room temperature while you cook the fish.

2. Season the mackerel fillets with salt and freshly ground black pepper, then grill them for 3-4 minutes on each side. Serve them on a bed of the tabbouleh.

Note: There has been some concern about the possible negative effect on the gut of the saponins that naturally coat and protect the quinoa seed. Just washing this layer off before use will eliminate the problem.

410 CALORIES

Chickpea, Coconut, and Cashew Curry

A creamy vegetarian curry with plenty of flavor, but not too spicy. Chickpeas contain a moderate amount of carbohydrates. They are also a good source of fiber and protein.

Serves 2 as a main dish
(4 as a side dish)

3 tbsp mild olive oil
   or rapeseed oil
1 onion, diced
2 celery stalks, diced
1 garlic clove, diced
¾ inch fresh ginger, grated
   or finely diced
1 tsp ground cumin
1 tsp mustard seeds
1 tsp ground turmeric
1 (14-oz) can chickpeas,
   rinsed and drained
¾ cup coconut milk
Juice of 1 lime
½ cup cashews
Large handful of fresh
   cilantro, chopped

•DAIRY-FREE
•GLUTEN-FREE
•GOOD FOR PHASE 1

1. Heat the oil in a pan and sauté the onion and celery for 4-5 minutes. Add the garlic, ginger, and spices and cook for 2 minutes longer.

2. Stir in the chickpeas, followed by the coconut milk, lime juice, and cashews, and simmer for 15-20 minutes.

3. Stir in the cilantro and season with salt and pepper before serving. This curry is delicious with Warm Red Rice Salad with Zucchini (page 90).

Tip: To cook chickpeas from scratch, cover them in 4 inches of water and soak them overnight, then boil them in a partially covered pot with three times the volume of water. Simmer for about 1 1/2 hours, or until they're tender, skimming off any foam on the surface.

710 CALORIES

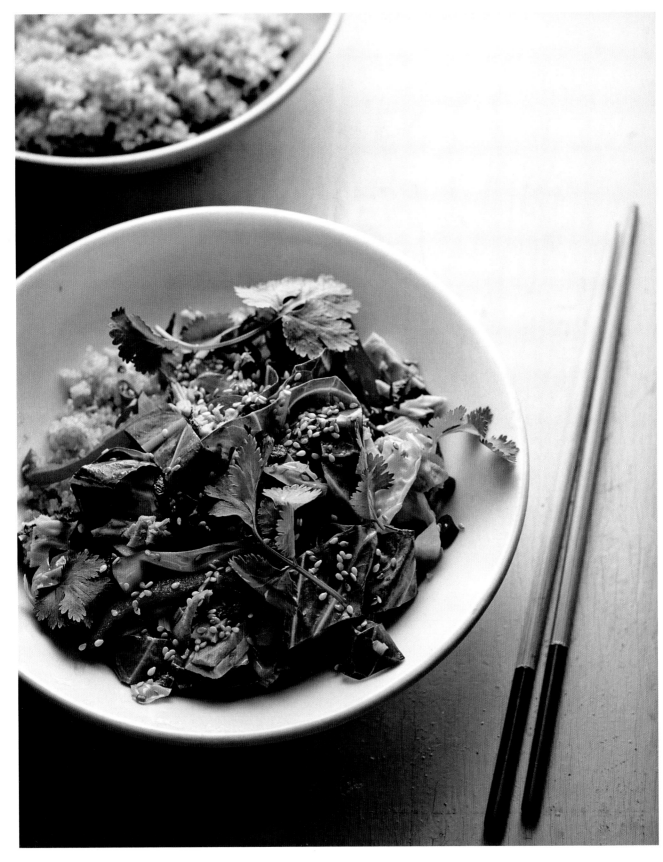

Tuna and Vegetable Stir-Fry with Seaweed

One of the easiest fish stir-fries you can make, conjured up with food from the pantry and vegetable drawer. What's more, it's bursting with omega-3 oils. We love it.

Serves 2

1 (6-oz) can tuna in oil, drained
1 tbsp fish sauce
1 tbsp rapeseed oil
1 small onion, sliced
1 red bell pepper, seeded and chopped
2 celery stalks, sliced
1½ cups shredded cabbage
½ inch fresh ginger, diced
1 garlic clove, sliced
½ red chile, seeded and diced, or ¼ tsp red pepper flakes
1½ nori seaweed sheets, chopped or shredded
1 tbsp rice wine

• DAIRY-FREE
• GLUTEN-FREE
• GOOD FOR PHASE 1

1. Place the tuna in a bowl and sprinkle the fish sauce over it. Leave it to stand.

2. Heat the oil in a wok and stir-fry the onion, bell pepper, and celery for 3-4 minutes. Add the cabbage, ginger, garlic, chile, and nori and continue to stir-fry for 1-2 minutes. Reduce the heat and add the rice wine, along with 1-2 tbsp water.

3. Gently stir in the tuna, without breaking it up too much, and simmer for a couple of minutes. Serve with Cauliflower Rice with Cilantro (page 174) or 2 tbsp brown basmati rice (add 100 calories).

Note: You may need to reduce the amount of onion, garlic, and bell pepper if you have IBS.

Tip: To add flavor and texture, scatter over 1-2 tsp toasted sesame seeds before serving.

580 CALORIES

Brazilian-Style Crab

Baked crab Brazilian-style, *casquinha de siri*, is a classic of the Bahia region, where the cooking often involves an exotic combination of Mediterranean and African ingredients. Crab is rich in high-quality protein.

Serves 4

1 tbsp olive oil

½ small onion, finely
    chopped

1 large garlic clove,
    chopped

1 red bell pepper, seeded
    and diced

8 oz white crab meat
    (fresh, canned, or frozen)

2 medium tomatoes, peeled,
    seeded, and chopped

½ cup coconut milk

Handful of fresh parsley,
    chopped

1 tbsp grated Parmesan
    (or vegan Parmesan)

Pinch of red pepper flakes
    or a few drops of Tabasco
    sauce, for serving

Wedges of lime, for serving

•DAIRY-FREE OPTION

•GLUTEN-FREE

•GOOD FOR PHASE 1

1. Preheat the oven to 350°F. Heat the oil in a saucepan and sauté the onion for 5 minutes. Add the garlic and bell pepper and cook for another 2-3 minutes, before adding the crab meat and tomatoes.

2. After 2 minutes, pour in the coconut milk, season with salt and pepper, and bring to a boil. Stir in the parsley and transfer the mixture to a baking dish. Sprinkle the Parmesan on top, and bake for 10-12 minutes, or until the top is golden.

3. Scatter over a few red pepper flakes, and serve alongside a bitter greens salad and some lime wedges.

370 CALORIES

Turmeric Coronation Chicken

An old British favorite given a healthy twist. Turmeric has been shown to have an impact on reducing inflammation, and possibly even the risk of cancer. The fat in the creamy sauce and the generous amount of black pepper in this recipe will significantly increase the beneficial effects of the curcumin in the turmeric.

Serves 2

2 tbsp olive oil

1 small onion, diced

2 celery stalks, diced

2 tbsp diced dried apricots

2 tsp ground turmeric

2 tsp curry powder

8 small cornichons, diced

1-2 tsp freshly ground
black pepper

6 oz cooked chicken
or turkey, chopped into
bite-size pieces

1¼ cups full-fat active
Greek-style yogurt (or
nondairy equivalent)

5 tbsp full-fat mayonnaise
(or nondairy equivalent)

Grated zest of 1 lime

2 tbsp chopped fresh
cilantro

⅓ cup slivered almonds,
toasted

•DAIRY-FREE OPTION

•GLUTEN-FREE

•GOOD FOR PHASE 1

1. Heat the oil in a pan and sauté the onion and celery for 4-5 minutes. Add the apricots, turmeric, and curry powder and cook for another 2-3 minutes, then set the mixture aside to cool.

2. Stir in the cornichons, pepper, chicken, yogurt, mayonnaise, lime zest, most of the cilantro, and half the almonds. Transfer the mixture to a bowl, then scatter the remaining cilantro and nuts on top.

3. Serve with brown rice (for 2 tbsp add 100 calories), Cauliflower Rice with Cilantro (page 174), or quinoa (for 2 tbsp add 120 calories) and a generous helping of a bitter greens salad such as arugula, watercress, and/or baby spinach.

720 CALORIES

Spinach Dal

This wonderful filling dal can be eaten on its own or as a side dish. Full of creamy, rich coconut flavors, it reheats well so you can keep it for a second hit later in the week. Lentils are generally great for your microbiome, being highly nutritious and containing a fair amount of protein.

Serves 4 as a main dish
(6-8 as a side dish)

3 tbsp olive oil or coconut
   oil
1 medium onion, chopped
2 garlic cloves, chopped
1 red chile, seeded and
   chopped, or ½ tsp
   red pepper flakes
1 tsp cumin seeds
1 tsp ground coriander
1 tsp ground turmeric
¾ inch fresh ginger, diced
Juice of ½ lemon
1 (14-oz) can coconut milk
1 (14-oz) can green lentils,
   rinsed and drained
3 cups spinach leaves
   (or kale, stems removed)
1 tbsp chopped fresh
   cilantro
8 oz paneer, chopped into
   ¾-inch cubes (optional)

•DAIRY-FREE OPTION
•GLUTEN-FREE

1. Heat the oil in a medium pan or casserole with a lid, and sauté the onion for 5 minutes. Stir in the garlic and cook for 1 more minute before adding the chile, spices, and ginger.

2. After 2 minutes, stir in the lemon juice, coconut milk, and lentils. Bring to a boil, then cover and allow to simmer for 10 minutes, stirring occasionally and adding more water if needed.

3. Add the spinach and cook for 3-5 minutes, then stir in the cilantro and season with salt and pepper. Scatter the paneer on top, if using. You might serve this dal with 1 tbsp Greek-style yogurt (add 75 calories) and Onion and Zucchini Bhajis (page 162).

Tips: Instead of lentils, you can use yellow split peas (chana dal), which take longer (35-40 minutes) to cook, or the smaller red lentils, which only take about 15 minutes, but give less texture. This dish freezes well and reheating it will increase the quantity of gut-friendly resistant starch, too.

Note: If you have IBS, reduce your portion size as the lentils can exacerbate symptoms.

570 CALORIES

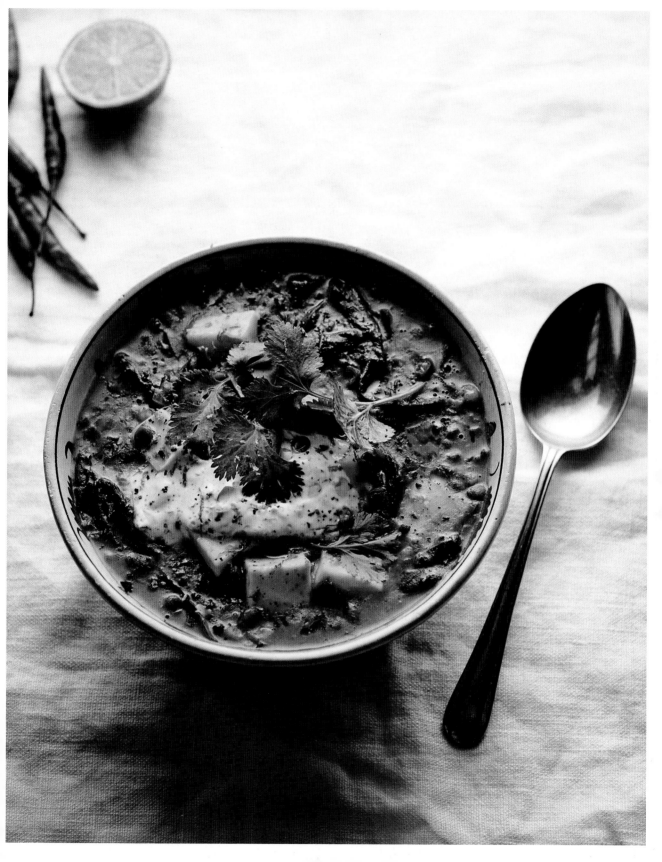

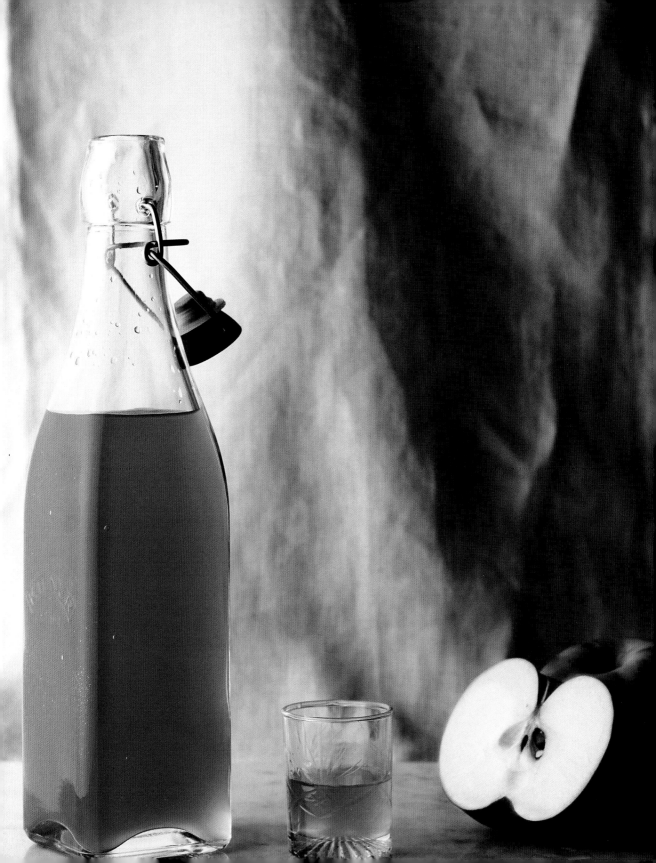

DRESSINGS AND FLAVORINGS

Dressings tend to be considered an afterthought, but in this book we have brought them center stage. They will transform a dull salad, add zip to the simplest of vegetables, and deliver lots of friendly bacteria to boost your biome.

Anchovy and Rosemary Dressing

Anchovies and rosemary make great companions in this lip-smacking dressing. It goes well with bitter greens and fish, and even makes a great sauce for roast beef or lamb, enhancing the flavors of the meat. Offers a good dose of healthy omega-3 fats, too.

Makes about ½ cup,
serves about 4

¼ cup extra-virgin olive oil

2 tsp rosemary leaves, very
  finely chopped

Juice of 1 lemon

5-6 salt-packed anchovies
  from a jar, finely chopped

1 tsp whole grain mustard

1 tsp honey

•DAIRY-FREE

•GLUTEN-FREE

•GOOD FOR PHASE 1

Whisk the oil, rosemary, lemon juice, and anchovies in a small bowl. Stir in the mustard and honey and season with freshly ground black pepper. Store in the fridge for up to a week.

Tip: As the anchovies are salty, there is no need to add salt to this dressing.

Lime Dressing

Citrus-scented and full of flavor, this dressing is great with any kind of fish.

Makes about ½ cup,
serves about 4

¼ cup olive oil

2 tbsp lime juice

½ tsp whole grain mustard

1 tsp finely chopped fresh
  mint, or 1 tbsp finely
  chopped fresh cilantro

•DAIRY-FREE

•GLUTEN-FREE

•GOOD FOR PHASE 1

Mix all the ingredients in a jar and store in the fridge for up to a week.

Salsa Verde with Seaweed

A super-healthy dressing that is wonderful to pour over fish or to add a bit of zing to vegetables or salads.

Makes about ½ cup,
serves about 4

3 anchovy fillets

3-4 tbsp chopped soft-leaf herbs, such as parsley, basil, oregano, and mint

1½ tbsp raw unfiltered apple cider vinegar

5 tbsp extra-virgin olive oil

1 garlic clove, crushed

1 tsp capers, rinsed

1 nori seaweed sheet, chopped (optional)

•DAIRY-FREE

•GLUTEN-FREE

•GOOD FOR PHASE 1

Blitz all the ingredients in a blender. Store the dressing in the fridge for up to a week.

Tip: Don't use too much mint, as it can overwhelm the other flavors. But a hint tastes great!

150 CALORIES

Apple Cider Vinegar Dressing

This classic dressing is sweet and tangy, and provides a great boost for your microbiome. Ideal to add to any bitter greens salad.

Makes about ½ cup,
serves about 6

½ cup extra-virgin olive oil

2 tbsp raw unfiltered apple cider vinegar

½ tbsp lemon juice

1 tsp maple syrup or honey

•DAIRY-FREE

•GLUTEN-FREE

•GOOD FOR PHASE 1

Mix all the ingredients in a jar and store in the fridge for up to a week.

140 CALORIES

Kefir and Buttermilk Dressings

Kefir is one of the best sources of probiotics you will find, as it contains complex, acid-tolerant bacteria that are able to make it down to your microbiome in beneficial numbers. And, as ever, homemade is the best (page 190). Buttermilk is the name given to a variety of traditional fermented milks found in the Middle East, Eastern Europe, Scandinavia, India, and other parts of Asia. In the US and Britain, buttermilk was originally made from the liquid left over after churning butter from cream. Choose buttermilk that states on the label that it has active cultures. These fermented milk dressings are all gluten-free, and are wonderfully enriching to almost any dish.

Lemony Buttermilk Dressing

A great dressing for salads and slaws. It delivers a double hit of different gut-friendly microbes from both the buttermilk and the preserved lemons.

Makes about 1 cup,
serves about 4

Generous ½ cup cultured
  buttermilk (or kefir)
½ tsp Colman's mustard
  powder
3 tbsp extra-virgin olive oil
½ tsp maple syrup
  (optional)
½ tbsp Preserved Lemons
  (page 184), finely diced
  (or grated zest and juice
  of ½ small lemon)
½ tsp xanthan gum
  (optional thickener)

Whisk the buttermilk and mustard in a bowl. Gradually add the oil, followed by the maple syrup (if using), preserved lemons, and xanthan gum, if using. Season well with sea salt and freshly ground black pepper.

70 CALORIES

Kefir Mustard Dressing

Makes about ¾ cup,
serves about 4
Generous ⅔ cup kefir
  (or cultured buttermilk)
2 tbsp extra-virgin olive oil
2 tsp whole grain mustard
½ tsp xanthan gum
  (optional thickener)

Whisk all the ingredients in a jar, season to taste, and store in the fridge for up to a week.

Creamy Pesto Kefir Dressing

A gutsy green dressing—and a great way to use up leftover Pistachio Pesto (page 99) and homemade Kefir Milk (page 190).

Makes about ¾ cup,
serves about 4
½ cup kefir (or cultured
  buttermilk)
2 tbsp Pistachio Pesto
1 tbsp grated Parmesan
½ tsp xanthan gum
  (optional thickener)

Whisk all the ingredients in a jar, season to taste, and store in the fridge for up to a week.

Turmeric Buttermilk Dressing

Makes about ¾ cup,
serves about 4
Generous ⅔ cup cultured
  buttermilk (or kefir)
Juice of ½ large lemon
2 tbsp olive oil
1 tsp Colman's mustard
  powder
1 tsp ground turmeric
½ tsp xanthan gum
  (optional thickener)

Whisk the buttermilk and lemon juice in a jar. Gradually whisk in the oil, mustard, turmeric, and xanthan gum, if using. Season to taste with sea salt and black pepper.

•ALL GLUTEN-FREE

Flavorings

The two mantras of the Clever Gut Diet are eat more vegetables and eat a greater variety of ingredients overall. These flavorings will have you longing for a plate of mixed vegetables to add them to. The butters can be stored in the freezer, ready to dollop on when you are ready. And the Nut Butter (page 123) will add protein and nutrients to all sorts of dishes, sweet and savory.

Dry Coconut Sambal

This Sri Lankan coconut mixture is full of good things, including turmeric, and can be guaranteed to spice things up. It's also a tasty way to enjoy some gut-friendly seaweed, though this is an optional addition.

Makes 6 tbsp
2 tsp ground turmeric (or fresh grated)
3 tbsp desiccated or shredded coconut
1 tbsp nam pla (Thai fish sauce)
1 tbsp tamari sauce (or soy sauce)
Juice of ½ lime
½-1 nori seaweed sheet, finely chopped (optional)
½ tsp red pepper flakes (optional)

•DAIRY-FREE
•GLUTEN-FREE
•GOOD FOR PHASE 1

Mix everything together. You can enhance the flavors by grinding the mixture in a mortar and pestle. Store in the fridge in a resealable jar for up to 2 weeks.

50 CALORIES PER TBSP SERVING

5 Flavored Butters

Allow the butter to soften at room temperature before beating it with the other ingredients. Chill it in the fridge for 10 minutes and then roll it into sausage shapes between sheets of parchment paper. Store in the fridge (up to 1 month) or freeze, then slice into disks to use.

Each makes 12 portions

Garlic and Parsley Butter

1 stick butter
3 garlic cloves, crushed
¼ cup finely chopped
    fresh parsley

Tip: Add 1 tsp dried or 2 tsp fresh tarragon and use it to baste or stuff a chicken.

Herb Butter

1 stick butter
3 tbsp finely chopped fresh
    herbs, such as thyme,
    oregano, or rosemary

Tip: You could also mash in ½ tbsp diced anchovies to jazz up cooked vegetables.

Whole Grain Mustard Butter

1 stick butter
1 tbsp whole grain mustard
1 garlic clove, crushed
1 tbsp capers, rinsed,
    drained, dried, and
    chopped

Tip: Dollop this butter on grilled or baked fish, or steaming-hot green vegetables.

Lemon and Pepper Butter

1 stick butter
Grated zest of 2 lemons
1 tbsp chopped fresh
    parsley
2 tsp freshly ground pink
    and black pepper

Tip: Delicious on fish or freshly steamed asparagus.

Blue Cheese Butter

1 stick butter
⅔ cup loosely packed
    crumbled blue cheese,
    such as Stilton or
    Roquefort

Tip: Top a cooked burger with this butter, and ditch the starchy bun.

•ALL GLUTEN-FREE

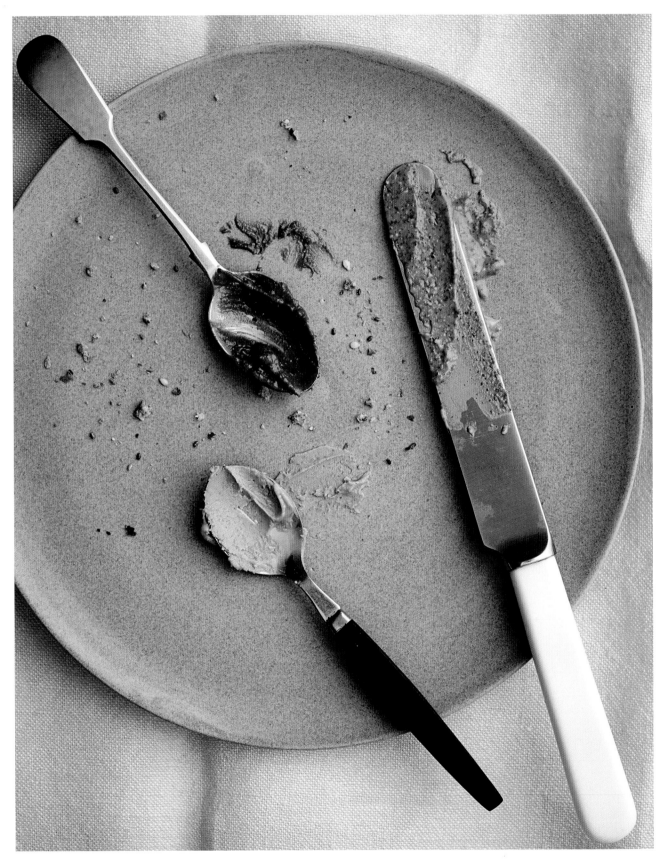

Nut Butter

There are myriad uses for nut butter, as well as eating it straight from the jar, as Michael sometimes does. Try spreading it on blinis or toast, baking with it, using it to thicken savory sauces or dips, or adding it to smoothies for extra protein. It's also delicious stirred into dressings.

Makes 1 small jar,
16 portions (each about
1 tbsp)

9 oz nuts, such as
  almonds, unsalted
  peanuts, macadamias,
  or cashews
1 tbsp coconut oil

•DAIRY-FREE
•GLUTEN-FREE
•GOOD FOR PHASE 1

1. Whizz the nuts to a fine powder in a blender or food processor. This can take 5-10 minutes, depending on the nuts used.

2. Add the coconut oil to loosen the mixture and whizz it again for up to 5 minutes, until it turns into a creamy paste.

3. Store in a resealable jar in the fridge for up to 4 weeks.

Tip: Using whole nuts, such as almonds with skin on rather than blanched, means all that fabulous fiber makes its way down the gut to boost your biome.

110 CALORIES

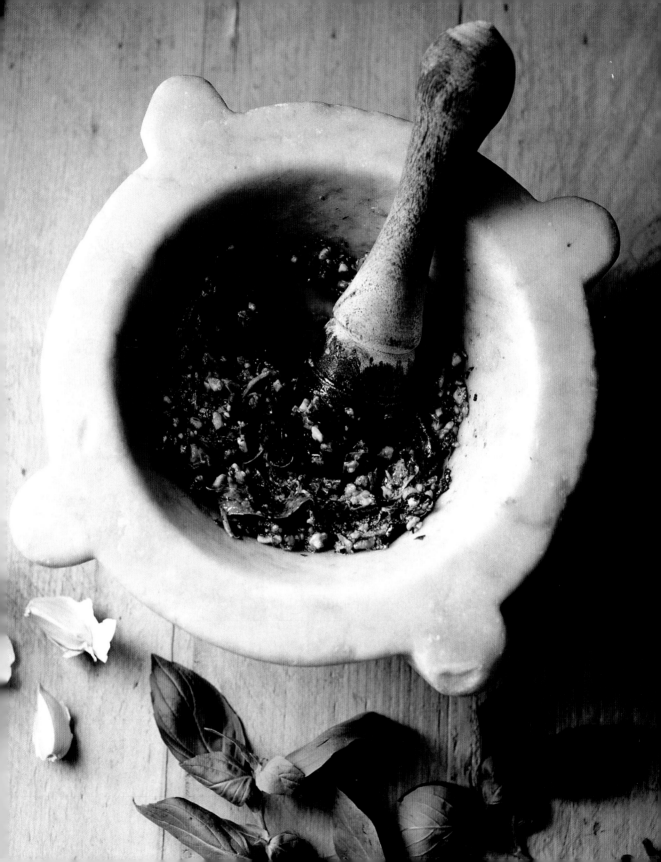

MAIN DISHES

It's best to eat most of your food earlier
in the day if you can—evidence shows
that you are less likely to store it as fat.
Try and do as the Mediterraneans do
and have your main meal at lunchtime,
followed by a light meal or snack
in the evening.

Poultry

Chicken and turkey are rich in protein. And birds raised with space to roam tend to contain more of the good stuff. Buy the best quality you can.

Baked Coconut Chicken Curry

This aromatic curry is bursting with goodness. Baking gives the chicken a delicious crispy skin.

Serves 4

Zest and juice of 2 limes
2 garlic cloves, diced
1 tsp ground turmeric
2 tsp medium curry powder
½ tsp cayenne pepper, or
   red pepper flakes to taste
   (optional)
4 large bone-in, skin-on
   chicken thighs
3 tbsp coconut oil, olive oil,
   or ghee
1 onion, diced
2 medium red bell
   peppers, seeded and
   sliced lengthwise
1 tbsp Thai fish sauce
   or soy sauce
¾ cup coconut milk
2 bay leaves
Generous handful of fresh
   cilantro, coarsely chopped

• DAIRY-FREE
• GLUTEN-FREE
• GOOD FOR PHASE 1

1. In a medium bowl, mix the lime zest and juice, garlic, turmeric, curry powder, and cayenne, if using. Coat the chicken in the mixture and season with salt and freshly ground black pepper. Let marinate for at least 1 hour or overnight in the fridge.

2. Preheat the oven to 350°F. Place a large casserole over medium heat, add the oil, and cook the onion and chicken, skin side down, for 4-5 minutes, or until the chicken skin is just turning golden brown. Turn them over and cook for 1-2 minutes more.

3. Reduce the heat and add any remaining marinade along with the bell peppers, fish sauce, coconut milk, and bay leaves. Bring everything to a simmer.

4. Place the casserole in the middle of the oven and bake for 25 minutes, basting the chicken occasionally, until it is cooked through. Remove from the oven, discard the bay leaves, and stir in the cilantro. Serve with a dollop of Greek-style yogurt (add 75 calories), 2 tbsp brown rice (add 100 calories), and a steamed green vegetable (add 20 calories).

880 CALORIES

Easy Chicken Tagine with Preserved Lemon

The North African equivalent of comfort food. Slow-cooked meat and vegetables are easier to digest, enabling you to absorb more nutrients, and leaving your digestive system with less work to do.

Serves 4

3 tbsp olive oil

1 large onion, diced

4 boneless, skinless chicken thighs (about 1⅓ lb)

2 garlic cloves, finely chopped

2 inches fresh ginger, peeled and diced

2 tsp ground cinnamon

2 tsp ground turmeric

2 tsp paprika

1¾ cups chicken stock

1 large red bell pepper, seeded and sliced

1 heaping tbsp diced Preserved Lemons (page 184), or ½ lemon (removed before serving)

⅔ cup dried apricots, halved

Generous handful of fresh cilantro, chopped

• DAIRY-FREE

• GLUTEN-FREE

• GOOD FOR PHASE 1

1. Preheat the oven to 300°F. Heat the oil in a medium casserole and sauté the onion for 2-3 minutes. Add the chicken and brown all over.

2. Stir in the garlic, ginger, and spices and cook for a couple more minutes. Pour in the stock, then add the bell pepper, preserved lemons, and apricots. Cover the casserole and bake, stirring occasionally, for 1-1½ hours, until the chicken is cooked through.

3. Stir the cilantro into the chicken tagine just before serving. Serve with 1 tbsp Greek-style yogurt (add 75 calories) and 2 tbsp brown rice (add 100 calories) or 2 tbsp quinoa (add 120 calories).

Tip: Ideally, use rice or quinoa that has been in the fridge or freezer for over 12 hours so that some of the starch is converted to more gut-friendly resistant starch.

470 CALORIES

Veira's Cilantro Chicken with Yogurt and Fennel

A light, tangy dish adapted from a recipe my mother learned while living in Malaysia.

Serves 4

2 garlic cloves, minced

1 inch fresh ginger, grated or finely chopped

Zest and juice of 2 limes

4 bone-in, skin-on chicken thighs (about 1¼ lb)

3 tbsp coconut or rapeseed oil

1 large onion, diced

Seeds from 6 cardamom pods

2 fennel bulbs, trimmed and quartered lengthwise

2 celery stalks, diced

1 tsp cornstarch

Large bunch of fresh cilantro, chopped

3 cups full-fat active Greek-style yogurt (or nondairy equivalent)

1 green chile, seeded and diced

•DAIRY-FREE OPTION

•GLUTEN-FREE

•GOOD FOR PHASE 1

1. In a nonmetallic bowl, mix the garlic, ginger, the lime zest, half the lime juice, salt, and pepper. Add the chicken and marinate in the fridge for at least 1 hour, or ideally overnight.

2. Preheat the oven to 350°F. Heat the oil in a large frying pan and sauté the chicken and onion over medium heat for 8-10 minutes, turning occasionally, until they are lightly golden. Add the cardamom seeds for the last 2 minutes of cooking. Spoon the contents into a large baking dish. Tuck the fennel and celery between the chicken pieces.

3. Pour the rest of the lime juice and any remaining marinade into the frying pan to deglaze it. Stir in the cornstarch and most of the cilantro, followed by the yogurt. Mix thoroughly, scraping the pan to incorporate all the chicken juices, then pour it over the chicken in the baking dish.

4. Cover the dish with a lid or foil and bake for 15 minutes. Uncover and bake for 15-20 minutes longer, until the chicken is slightly browned and cooked through. Before serving, scatter some green chile and the remaining cilantro on top.

5. This goes well with Cauliflower Rice with Cilantro (page 174) and stir-fried greens (add 40 calories). For an extra yogurt kick, mix 1 cup Greek-style yogurt with 1 tbsp cilantro and 1 tbsp lime juice and dollop it on top.

650 CALORIES

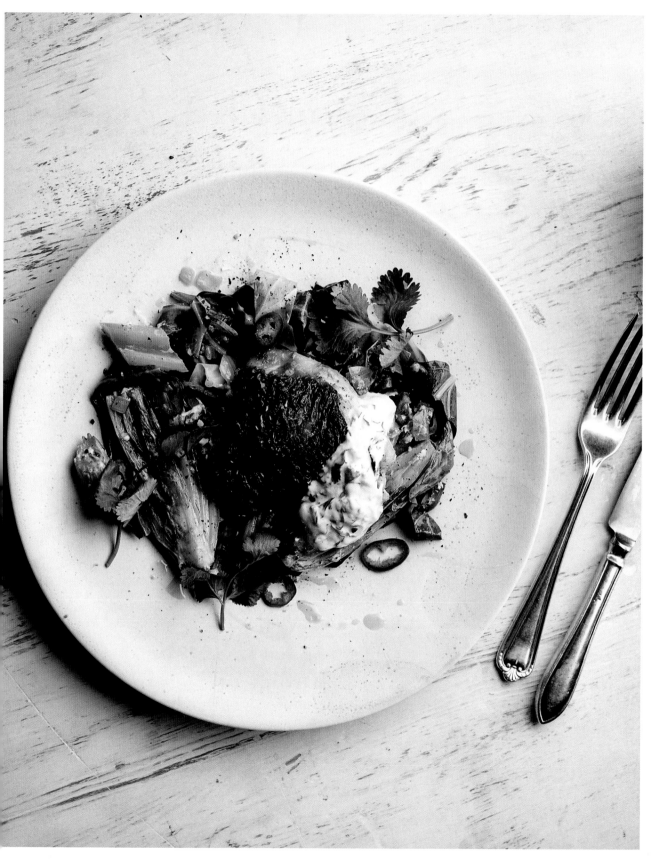

Lazy Lemon and Lime Chicken

We have cooked many versions of this dish over the years and love the way the flavors are lifted by the preserved lemon. It is easy to preserve your own and they taste so much better than the stuff you can buy.

Serves 4

Juice of 2 limes

2 garlic cloves, crushed

1½ tsp thyme leaves

1 tsp red pepper flakes

4 boneless, skin-on chicken thighs

3 tbsp olive oil

4 oz mushrooms, sliced

2 medium onions, sliced

1 Preserved Lemon (page 184), cut into wedges

1 cup mixed red and white quinoa, or gluten-free bulgur wheat and quinoa

1¾ cups hot chicken stock

•DAIRY-FREE

•GLUTEN-FREE

•GOOD FOR PHASE 1

1. Make a marinade with the lime juice, garlic, thyme, and red pepper flakes. Pour it over the chicken in a nonmetallic bowl and marinate for 1 hour, or up to 12 hours in the fridge.

2. Heat the oil in a frying pan and brown the chicken all over. Meanwhile, spread the mushrooms, onions, and preserved lemon wedges over the bottom of a flameproof casserole or large saucepan. Sprinkle over the quinoa, then place the browned chicken on top.

3. Use half the stock to deglaze the frying pan and pour it over the chicken. Then add the remaining stock.

4. Simmer over low heat for 35-40 minutes, checking from time to time that the quinoa has not absorbed all the stock, and add a little water if necessary. Serve with a vegetable of your choice, such as grilled zucchini slices or steamed kale (add 20 calories).

560 CALORIES

Turkey and Mushroom Bolognese

Two great base ingredients here: Turkey, which offers a nice alternative to beef, cooks more quickly and makes a really tasty Bolognese. Mushrooms, which are incredibly low in carbohydrates and full of gut-friendly fiber, have a texture that is almost like meat. We love them both.

Serves 4

¼ cup olive oil

1 large red onion, diced

1 garlic clove, crushed

1 lb cremini mushrooms, thinly sliced

10 oz ground turkey

2 (14-oz) cans diced tomatoes

2 medium carrots, grated

2 bay leaves

1 tsp dried mixed herbs

1 lb spiralized butternut squash or zucchini, for serving

•DAIRY-FREE

•GLUTEN-FREE

•GOOD FOR PHASE 1

1. Heat the oil in a large skillet and sauté the onion for 5-6 minutes. Add the garlic and mushrooms and cook for 3-4 minutes, stirring occasionally.

2. Stir in the turkey and cook for 4-5 minutes, then add the tomatoes, carrots, bay leaves, and herbs. Season with salt and pepper, and simmer for about 20 minutes. Discard the bay leaves.

3. Meanwhile, steam the spiralized squash. Divide it among 4 warmed plates, top with the Bolognese, and serve.

510 CALORIES

Fish

One of the healthiest foods on the planet, fish is loaded with important nutrients that most of us don't get enough of. Try to eat fish at least twice a week, choosing responsibly sourced varieties where possible.

Baked Salmon with Seaweed Pesto

A classic recipe for baked salmon, enhanced by the delicious umami flavors of gut-friendly, nutrient-packed seaweed.

Serves 4

3 red bell peppers, seeded and cut into large pieces

2 medium zucchini, sliced

2 red onions, cut into wedges

2 tbsp olive oil

¼ cup pesto (page 99)

1½ nori seaweed sheets, chopped

4 (5-oz) salmon fillets

• DAIRY-FREE

• GLUTEN-FREE

• GOOD FOR PHASE 1

1. Preheat the oven to 350°F. Place the bell peppers, zucchini, and onions in a large roasting pan, toss with the oil, and bake for 12-15 minutes.

2. Meanwhile, combine the pesto and nori and spread over the salmon fillets.

3. Place the salmon on top of the roasted vegetables and cover the pan with foil. Bake for 15 minutes, or until the salmon is no longer translucent, removing the foil for the last 5 minutes (don't overcook the salmon as it will dry out).

4. Serve with a leafy green salad. It works well drizzled with Creamy Pesto Kefir Dressing (page 119).

540 CALORIES

Mackerel Fillets with Spiced Coconut

Mackerel is a great value, and provides more omega-3 oils than almost any other fish. The tangy flavors in this crispy sambal topping really pep it up.

Serves 2
2 small mackerel fillets
1 egg white
2 tbsp Dry Coconut Sambal
  (page 120)
Juice of ½ lime

•DAIRY-FREE
•GLUTEN-FREE
•GOOD FOR PHASE 1

1. Place the mackerel fillets skin side down in a lightly greased baking dish.

2. In a small bowl, lightly whisk the egg white, then stir in the sambal and season with salt and pepper. Spread the mixture over the fillets and marinate in the fridge for up to 2 hours, if possible.

3. Preheat the oven to 325°F. Bake the fillets for 12-15 minutes, or until the surface becomes crisp. Squeeze the lime juice over the fish. Serve with cooked quinoa (for 2 tbsp add 120 calories) and Scorched Purple Radicchio (page 160).

510 CALORIES

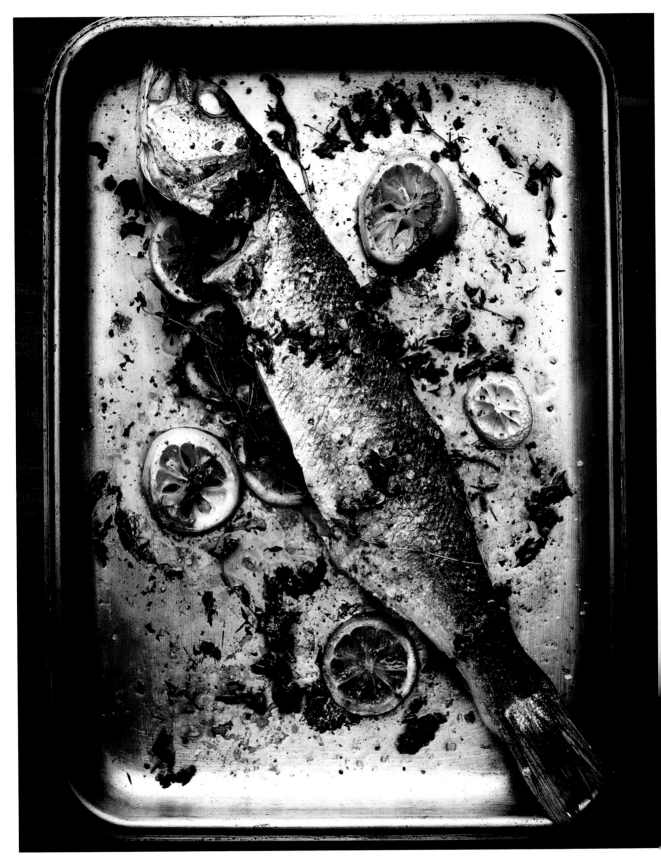

Sea Bass with Seaweed Salsa Verde

Crisp, succulent, and full of flavors of the sea. A delicious way to boost your omega-3s and treat your microbiome to some seaweed.

Serves 2

1 tbsp olive or rapeseed oil

2 sea bass fillets

Salsa Verde with Seaweed
   (page 117)

•DAIRY-FREE

•GLUTEN-FREE

•GOOD FOR PHASE 1

1. Place a frying pan over medium heat, add the oil, and cook the fillets skin side up for 4-5 minutes.

2. Turn the fillets over and drizzle with half the salsa verde. Cook for 3-4 minutes longer, until the fillets are no longer translucent. Transfer to a plate and pour over the rest of the salsa.

3. Serve with 3-4 small boiled potatoes (ideally reheated so they contain more resistant starch; add 40 calories) and Pea and Edamame Mash (page 162).

Tip: If using a whole fish, stuff some Seaweed Salsa Verde into the cavity for extra flavor.

380 CALORIES

Sweet Potato, Kale, and Cod Fishcakes

These Moroccan-flavored fishcakes can also be made with other fish, such as salmon or trout. The sweet potatoes help bind them and are easy on the gut. They are delicious served with a crunchy green salad, or Green Beans and Edamame with Anchovies (page 87), or even for breakfast, topped with a poached egg. You might also serve them with Creamy Nutmeg Spinach (page 160) and Puy Lentils with Balsamic Vinegar (page 169).

Serves 4

1½ lb sweet potatoes, peeled and chopped

1 cup shredded kale

3 spring onions, finely chopped

1 tsp harissa paste

1 egg, beaten

10 oz cod fillet

3 tbsp buckwheat flour

2 tbsp olive oil

•DAIRY-FREE

•GLUTEN-FREE

•GOOD FOR PHASE 1

1. Steam the sweet potatoes for 6 minutes, then add the kale and steam for another 6-8 minutes, or until the potatoes are tender. Transfer the vegetables to a bowl and lightly mash with a fork or potato masher. Add the onions, harissa, and egg and season well with salt and black pepper.

2. Meanwhile, place the cod in a pan and cover with water. Bring to a simmer and cook for 4-5 minutes, until the flesh flakes away from the skin easily. Add the flaked fish to the vegetables, stirring well with a fork to mix all the ingredients together. With wet hands, form the mixture into 8 patties. Dust them with a little flour and chill in the fridge for 20 minutes.

3. Heat the oil in a frying pan over medium heat and cook the fishcakes for 3-4 minutes on each side, or until golden.

340 CALORIES

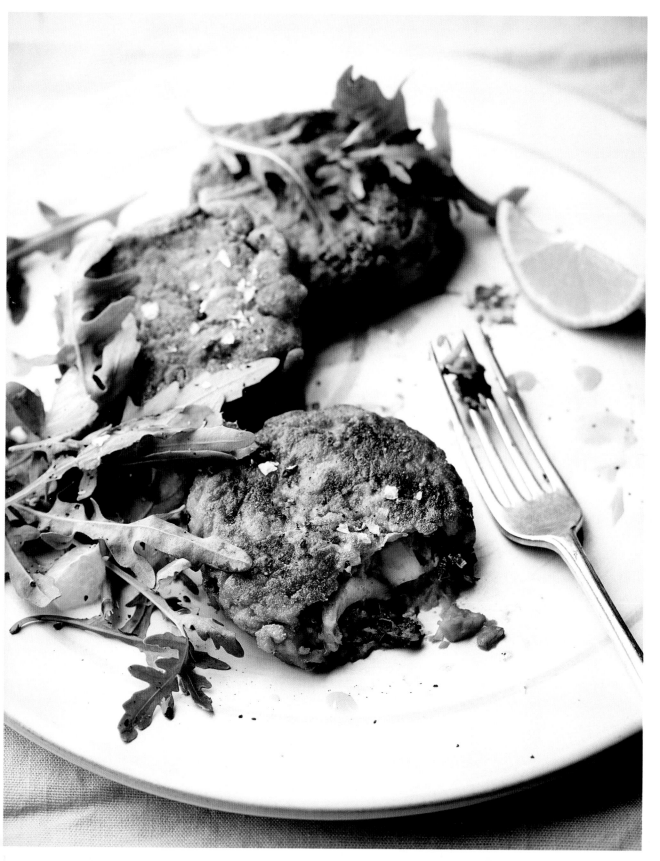

Seafood

You will have noticed that nearly all of our fish and seafood recipes contain seaweed. It is not key to the dishes, so it can be reduced or left out altogether if you prefer. But sprinkle it on liberally if you can. It adds a wonderful salty, seafoody taste and your microbiome thrives on it.

Shrimp with Pasta and Seaweed

We love shrimp and it works brilliantly in this easy Mediterranean-style pasta dish.

Serves 2

8 oz whole wheat (or gluten-free) pasta

¼ cup olive oil

2 celery stalks, diced

½ fennel bulb, sliced

4 spring onions, trimmed and sliced

2 garlic cloves, diced

¾ oz anchovies (or to taste), drained and chopped

½ tsp dried thyme

12 oz cooked shrimp

⅔ (10-oz) package frozen spinach, thawed

2 nori seaweed sheets, finely chopped

Juice of 1 lemon

¼ tsp Tabasco sauce, or to taste

•DAIRY-FREE

•GLUTEN-FREE OPTION

•GOOD FOR PHASE 1

1. Cook the pasta according to the package instructions.

2. Meanwhile, in a large deep frying pan, heat the oil and sauté the celery, fennel, onions, and garlic for 4-5 minutes, until they're soft but not brown. Add the anchovies and thyme and cook for a couple of minutes.

3. Add the shrimp, spinach, and nori, along with the lemon juice, Tabasco, salt, and black pepper.

4. Add the drained pasta to the pan, tossing it well to coat it with the sauce. Serve with Pea and Edamame Mash (page 162) or a multicolored salad (add 20 calories).

840 CALORIES

Seafood with Seaweed Risotto

We recommend eating lots of different kinds of seafood—and this risotto gives you the opportunity to do just that. You can buy frozen seafood mixes, containing shrimp, squid, mussels, surimi, and/or other seafood, in large supermarkets and warehouse stores.

Serves 2

3 cups vegetable stock

3 tbsp olive oil

1 small onion, diced

1 large garlic clove, chopped

1¼ cups brown rice

1 (14-16-oz) package frozen mixed seafood, thawed

½ cup white wine

Juice of 1 lemon

2 tbsp chopped fresh parsley

1½ nori seaweed sheets, chopped

2 tbsp grated Parmesan (or vegan Parmesan)

½ tsp red pepper flakes (optional)

•DAIRY-FREE OPTION

•GLUTEN-FREE

•GOOD FOR PHASE 1

1. Bring the stock to a simmer in a saucepan.

2. Heat 2 tbsp of the oil in another larger saucepan and sauté the onions and garlic for 3-4 minutes, or until they start to soften. Add the rice and stir for a couple of minutes, then pour over enough stock to cover it. Leave it to simmer, covered, stirring occasionally and adding more stock as the rice absorbs it.

3. When the rice has been cooking for around 10 minutes, heat the remaining 1 tbsp oil in a frying pan and stir-fry the seafood for 2-3 minutes, then spoon it into the risotto.

4. Deglaze the frying pan with the wine, then pour it into the risotto. Continue to cook and stir, adding stock, for about 30 minutes, by which time the rice should be cooked al dente. In the last few minutes of cooking stir in the lemon juice, parsley, seaweed, Parmesan, and red pepper flakes, if using.

5. Serve with a bitter greens salad (page 56) or cooked greens (add 20 calories).

560 CALORIES

shrimp are high in protein, low in calories, and a good source of vitamin D, vitamin B12, iron, and selenium.

Thai Shrimp with Coconut Milk and Seaweed

Simple to make and packed with health-boosting antioxidants.

Serves 2

5 oz green-pea pasta
  (or whole wheat pasta)
2 cups broccoli florets
3 tbsp coconut oil
½ red onion, sliced
¾ inch fresh ginger, grated
½ red chile, seeded and
  finely chopped, or ¼ tsp
  red pepper flakes
¾ cup coconut milk
Juice of 1 lime
½ tbsp Thai fish sauce
2 nori seaweed sheets,
  chopped
8 oz shrimp, peeled and
  deveined
Generous handful of fresh
  cilantro, chopped

•DAIRY-FREE
•GLUTEN-FREE
•GOOD FOR PHASE 1

1. Cook the pasta according to the package instructions.

2. Steam the broccoli for 4-5 minutes and set aside.

3. Heat the oil in a large frying pan and sauté the onion for 4-5 minutes. Add the ginger and chile, cook for 1 minute, and then pour in the coconut milk, lime juice, fish sauce, seaweed, and shrimp.

4. Bring to a simmer, then add the broccoli and cook for 2 minutes more, or until the shrimp are cooked through. Stir in the pasta with the cilantro and serve.

700 CALORIES

Squid Provençal

This makes a gorgeous, deep-red, herby stew. Squid is a good value, and an excellent source of protein.

Serves 2

3 tbsp olive oil

1 small onion, sliced

1 red bell pepper, seeded
and finely diced

2 garlic cloves, finely
chopped

1 tsp thyme, fresh or dried

2 bay leaves

1 (14-oz) can diced
tomatoes

½ cup white wine

½ tsp red pepper flakes

10 oz cleaned squid
(thawed frozen is fine)

Handful of fresh parsley
or cilantro, chopped,
for serving

•DAIRY-FREE

•GLUTEN-FREE

•GOOD FOR PHASE 1

1. Heat the oil in a pan and sauté the onion, bell pepper, and garlic for 3-4 minutes. Add the thyme and bay leaves, along with the tomatoes, wine, and red pepper flakes, and simmer for 10 minutes.

2. Turn the heat down as low as you can, add the squid, and simmer or place the pan in a 200°F oven, covered, for about 50 minutes. Don't actually boil it as it will become rubbery. Discard the bay leaves.

3. To thicken the sauce, remove 1-2 cupfuls of it with a ladle and blitz it in a blender, then return it to the pan. Garnish with the parsley. Serve the stew with 2 tbsp brown rice (ideally cooled and reheated to increase resistant starch; add 100 calories) or quinoa (add 120 calories) and a multicolored leafy salad (add 20 calories).

430 CALORIES

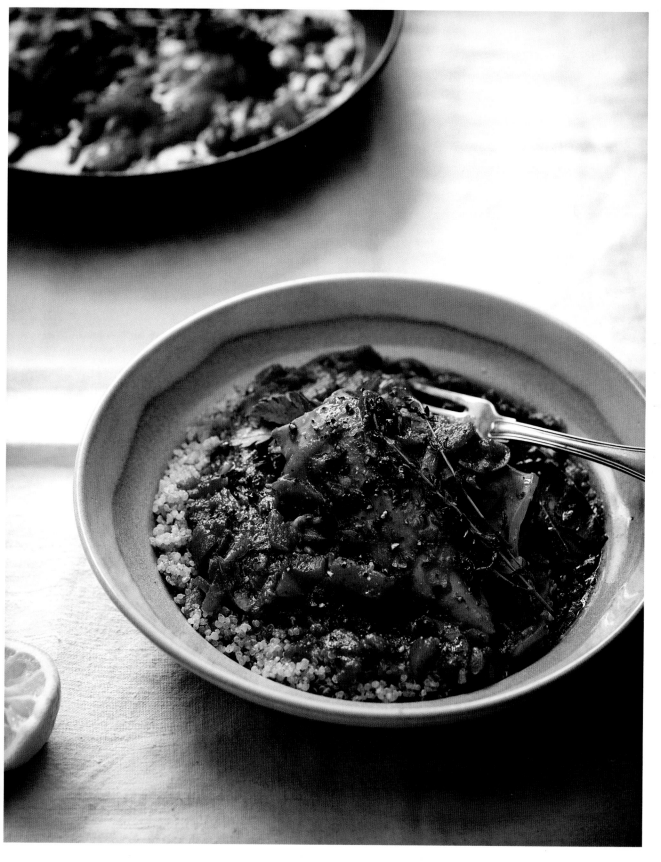

Vegetarian Dishes

There are many quick vegetarian dishes elsewhere in this book. These recipes take a bit longer to prepare but are definitely worth the effort.

Marinated Tofu Stir-Fry with Noodles

Marinating and then baking tofu transforms it from something pale and rather bland into a flavorsome delicacy—so tasty you could nibble it on its own.

Serves 2

2 tbsp tamari sauce (or soy sauce)
1 garlic clove, crushed
2 tsp sesame oil (optional)
¾ inch fresh ginger, diced
8 oz silken tofu, drained and chopped into ½-inch pieces
4 oz soba noodles (or gluten-free alternative)
2 tbsp coconut oil
1 red bell pepper, seeded and chopped
4 spring onions, sliced
1½ cups chopped tender broccoli or broccolini
¾ cup vegetable stock
2 tbsp cashews
5 oz bean sprouts
½ tsp red pepper flakes (optional)

• DAIRY-FREE
• GLUTEN-FREE OPTION
• GOOD FOR PHASE 1

1. Preheat the oven to 325°F and line a baking sheet with parchment paper.

2. In a medium bowl, mix the tamari, garlic, sesame oil, and ginger. Gently toss the tofu in the marinade, then spread it on the baking sheet and season with black pepper.

3. Bake the tofu for 30 minutes, turning it once halfway through cooking. It should be golden and crisp at the edges.

4. Cook the noodles in a pan of boiling water for 5 minutes or according to the package instructions. Drain and refresh under cold running water.

5. Heat the coconut oil in a wok over medium-high heat, and stir-fry the bell pepper, onions, and broccoli for 2-3 minutes. Reduce the heat and add ¼ cup of the stock. Continue to stir-fry for 3-4 minutes, then add the tofu, cashews, bean sprouts, and red pepper flakes. Pour in the remaining stock with the noodles, bring to a simmer, and serve immediately.

410 CALORIES

Vegetable and Paneer Curry

An easy vegetarian curry with lots of flavor that's not too spicy.

Serves 4

2 eggplant, diced

2 red bell peppers, seeded
   and diced

½ small cauliflower, broken
   into florets

6 tbsp mild olive oil or
   rapeseed oil

2 onions, 1 sliced into rings
   and 1 diced

¾ inch fresh ginger,
   chopped

2 garlic cloves, chopped

1 tsp mustard seeds

1 tsp ground turmeric

1 tsp cumin seeds

½-1 tsp red pepper flakes

1 (14-oz) can diced
   tomatoes

1 cup vegetable stock

6 oz paneer or tofu, sliced

Handful of fresh cilantro,
   chopped

•DAIRY-FREE OPTION

•GLUTEN-FREE

•GOOD FOR PHASE 1

1. Preheat the oven to 400°F. Spread the eggplant, bell peppers, and cauliflower in a roasting pan. Drizzle with 2 tbsp of the oil and season with a pinch of salt. Bake the vegetables for 15-20 minutes, or until they start to caramelize, turning them once.

2. Heat 2 tbsp of the oil in a frying pan and fry the onion rings, stirring frequently, until they're crisp and golden brown. Set them aside.

3. Heat the remaining 2 tbsp oil in a medium casserole and sauté the diced onions for 4-5 minutes before adding the ginger, garlic, and spices. Cook for 2 more minutes.

4. Remove the vegetables from the oven and spoon them into the casserole, stirring to give them a good coating of the spice mixture. Pour in the diced tomatoes and stock and bring to a boil. Reduce the heat and simmer for 15-20 minutes. Stir in the paneer cheese during the last 5 minutes. Season to taste with salt and black pepper and stir in most of the cilantro. Scatter the rest over the top, along with the sautéed onion rings.

5. Serve with Cauliflower Rice with Cilantro (page 174) or 2 tbsp brown basmati rice (100 calories), 1 tbsp Greek-style yogurt (75 calories), and Onion and Zucchini Bhajis (page 162).

430 CALORIES

In addition to being high in gut-friendly soluble fiber, black beans contain significant levels of phytonutrients—especially flavonoids, the antioxidants found most commonly in deeply colored foods.

Black Bean Beet Burgers

These burgers look so like beef burgers they are in danger of putting off vegetarians. A seeded bun makes them a real treat.

Serves 4 (2 burgers each)
5 oz beets, peeled and diced into ¼-inch pieces
1 small onion, finely diced
½ tsp ground cumin
1 tsp ground coriander
3 tbsp olive oil
1 (14-oz) can black beans (or kidney beans), drained but not rinsed
1 large garlic clove, crushed
½ tsp red pepper flakes
Zest of 2 limes
1 medium egg, beaten
¾ cup cooked quinoa (red, white, or black)
⅓ cup grated vegan Parmesan
2 tbsp chopped fresh parsley

•DAIRY-FREE
•GLUTEN-FREE
•GOOD FOR PHASE 1

1. Preheat the oven to 350°F. Mix the beets and onion in a medium bowl with the cumin, coriander, 1 tbsp of the oil, the salt, and black pepper. Spoon the mixture into a roasting pan and bake, covered, for 20-25 minutes, until the beets start to soften.

2. Meanwhile, place the beans, garlic, red pepper flakes, and lime zest in the bowl used for the beets. Season with salt and black pepper and mash with a fork or a hand blender, leaving some texture.

3. When the beets are cooked, allow them to cool for 10 minutes before mixing into the beans. Then add the egg, quinoa, Parmesan, and parsley and mix thoroughly. With wet hands, shape the mixture into 8 medium patties. Chill in the fridge for 20 minutes.

4. Heat the remaining 2 tbsp oil in a frying pan and cook the burgers over medium heat for 5-6 minutes on each side. Serve on a whole grain bun (add 100 calories) or Whole Grain Flatbread (page 195), with Pickled Zucchini (page 188) or Red Cabbage Sauerkraut (page 185), or on a plate with 2 tbsp bulgur wheat (add 100 calories) or quinoa (add 120 calories) and Bitter Greens and Toasted Pine Nut Salad (page 56).

Note: If you have IBS, eat beans in moderation and avoid during the first two weeks of Phase 1 as beans can exacerbate symptoms.

280 CALORIES W/O THE BUN

Quorn and Parsnip Shepherd's Pie

Quorn is made from mycoprotein, a fungus grown in a fermentation process similar to that used in the production of yogurt, and is an excellent source of protein, fiber, and nutrients. For a non-vegetarian version, use ground turkey or pork instead.

Serves 4

10 oz parsnips, scrubbed and diced into ¾-inch cubes

10 oz celeriac, scrubbed and diced into ¾-inch cubes

5 tbsp olive oil

1 onion, diced

2 bay leaves

1 tsp ground cumin

1 tsp ground cinnamon

1 (12-oz) package Quorn grounds

5 oz butternut squash, peeled and diced

1 (14-oz) can diced tomatoes

1 tbsp raw unfiltered apple cider vinegar

1 vegetable bouillon cube

2 tbsp grated Parmesan (or vegan Parmesan)

3 cups fresh spinach, chopped

•DAIRY-FREE OPTION

•GLUTEN-FREE

•GOOD FOR PHASE 1

1. Preheat the oven to 350°F. Cook the parsnips and celeriac in a pan of simmering salted water for 15-18 minutes, or until they're soft.

2. Meanwhile, in a large casserole with a lid, heat 3 tbsp of the oil and sauté the onion for 5 minutes, adding the bay leaves and spices halfway through. Add the Quorn and cook for 5-7 minutes, stirring frequently. Mix in the butternut squash along with the tomatoes, vinegar, ¾ cup water, and the crumbled bouillon cube. Cover and simmer for about 10 minutes. Season with salt and pepper. Discard the bay leaves.

3. Drain the parsnip and celeriac, return to the pan, and mash vigorously with 1 tbsp of the oil and 1 tbsp Parmesan. Layer the spinach on top of the Quorn mixture, followed by the mash. Scatter the rest of the Parmesan on top and drizzle over the remaining 1 tbsp oil.

4. Bake in the middle of the oven for 25-30 minutes, or until the pie is golden brown on top. Serve with steamed greens (add 20 calories).

410 CALORIES

Red Meat

Red meat is fine for you in modest amounts and is an excellent source of protein and iron. We are gradually moving toward having red meat only about twice a week. The upside of this is that we find we are enjoying our vegetables more, both incorporated into the main dish and as sides. In many of these dishes the vegetables contribute vital taste, texture, and flavor.

Prosciutto-Wrapped Pork Loin

The prosciutto and cream cheese wrapping keeps the pork moist and succulent, and the roasted fennel adds a delicious sweetness.

Serves 4

5 oz cream cheese

2 garlic cloves, finely chopped

2 tsp chopped fresh oregano, or 1 tsp dried

1 lb pork loin

5 slices of prosciutto or serrano ham

2 fennel bulbs, trimmed and quartered

2 tbsp olive oil

•DAIRY-FREE OPTION

•GLUTEN-FREE

•GOOD FOR PHASE 1

1. Preheat the oven to 350°F. Mix the cream cheese, garlic, oregano, and some salt and black pepper. Spread the mixture over the pork loin and then wrap the prosciutto around it, covering as much as possible.

2. Place the pork in a roasting pan with the fennel quarters and drizzle with the oil. Bake for 30-35 minutes, basting occasionally. It is cooked when the juices run clear.

3. Serve it sliced, with 2 tbsp quinoa (add 120 calories) and a large helping of dark greens, such as kale, Swiss chard, or spring greens (add 20 calories). Or add some Eggplant Chips (page 175).

Tip: For a nondairy version, you can substitute the cream cheese with hummus.

420 CALORIES

Beef and Orange Stew with Mushrooms

The best of comfort food. Slow-cooked and gentle on the gut. Lots of lovely mushrooms, too!

Serves 2

3 tbsp olive oil

1 large white onion, diced

10 oz stew beef, diced

1 inch fresh ginger, diced

2 bay leaves

1 star anise (optional)

1 cup passata (or strained crushed tomatoes)

1 tbsp raw unfiltered apple cider vinegar

2 tsp Dijon mustard

Zest and juice of 1 orange

3 large celery stalks, diced

1 carrot, diced

1 organic beef or vegetarian bouillon cube

7 oz mushrooms, sliced

• DAIRY-FREE

• GLUTEN-FREE

• GOOD FOR PHASE 1

1. Preheat the oven to 325°F. Heat the oil in a large casserole and sauté the onion for 5 minutes. Add the meat and brown all over. Add the ginger, bay leaves, star anise (if using), passata, vinegar, mustard, and orange zest and juice and mix well.

2. Add the celery and carrot, then crumble in the bouillon cube. Add just enough water to cover everything. Stir gently, bring to a simmer, and cover the casserole. Bake for 2-2½ hours, adding the mushrooms after 1 hour. The stew is done when the meat is tender. Check from time to time and add more water if needed. Discard the bay leaves. Season to taste with salt and black pepper.

3. Serve with greens, such as steamed kale or broccoli (add 20 calories), and 3-4 small new potatoes (add 40 calories).

700 CALORIES

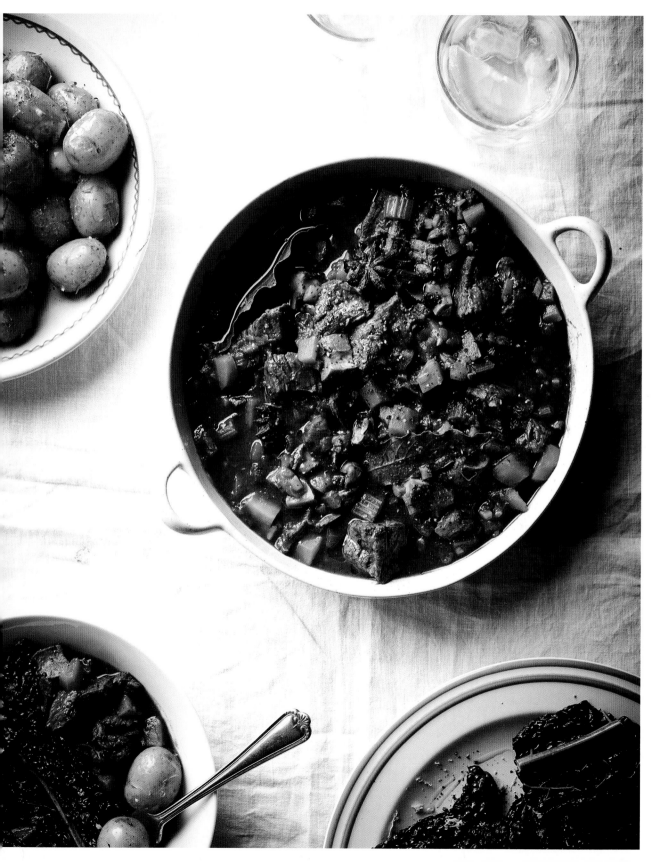

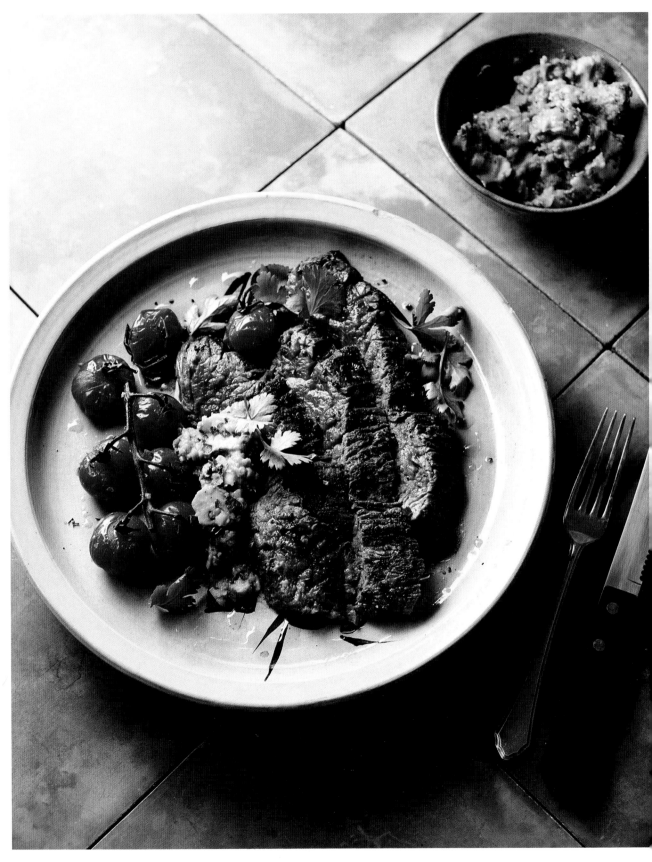

Steak with Guacamole and Blistered Tomatoes

Pounding the steak before you cook it, particularly if it's an economic cut or is fairly thick, will tenderize it and make it easier to digest. Marinating it, especially in an acidic element such as lemon juice, will aid this process, and also enhance the flavor.

Serves 2

2 (4-oz) steaks, skirt
  or sirloin
1 tsp ground cumin
1 garlic clove, crushed
1 tbsp lemon juice
1 tbsp olive oil
1 avocado, diced
½ red onion, diced
½-1 tsp red pepper flakes
1 tbsp chopped fresh
  cilantro or basil
1 tbsp lime juice
16 cherry tomatoes, halved

•DAIRY-FREE

•GLUTEN-FREE

•GOOD FOR PHASE 1

1. If using thick steaks, place on a cutting board and pound them with the rough side of a mallet. If you don't have a mallet you can use the end of a wooden rolling pin. Bash from the middle outward. Don't pound too hard or you will shred the meat.

2. In a bowl, mix the cumin, garlic, lemon juice, and oil. Place the steaks in a shallow dish and pour the mixture over them (turning them to make sure they are well covered). Marinate for 20 minutes.

3. Meanwhile, make the guacamole by mashing together the avocado, onion, red pepper flakes, cilantro, and lime juice. Season with salt and pepper and set aside.

4. Heat a grill pan or frying pan over high heat. Cook the tomatoes, cut side up, for 3-4 minutes, until the skins are blistered. Remove from the pan and add the steaks. Cook for about 3 minutes on each side (for a medium steak).

5. Slice up the steaks, top with the blistered tomatoes, and serve the guacamole on the side.

470
CALORIES

Sausage and Mediterranean Sheet Pan Bake

Cooked all on one baking sheet, and containing lots of fiber-rich vegetables.

Serves 2

4 good-quality free-range
sausages (or gluten-free)

1 red bell pepper, seeded
and sliced

1 yellow bell pepper,
seeded and sliced

1 medium red onion,
cut into 8 wedges

3 tbsp olive oil

1 tsp dried thyme
or oregano

1 medium zucchini,
cut into batons

4 oz cherry tomatoes
(preferably on the vine)

1½ tbsp balsamic vinegar

2 heaping tbsp cooked
whole grains (quinoa,
bulgur wheat, or pearl
barley)

•DAIRY-FREE

•GLUTEN-FREE OPTION

•GOOD FOR PHASE 1

1. Preheat the oven to 350°F. Place the sausages in a large roasting pan with the bell peppers and onion. Drizzle over the oil, and sprinkle the herbs, some Maldon sea salt, and freshly ground black pepper on top.

2. Place the pan in the center of the oven and bake for 15 minutes. Stir in the zucchini and tomatoes and drizzle over the balsamic vinegar. Return the pan to the oven and bake for 10-15 minutes, or until the sausages start to brown and are cooked through.

3. Stir in the whole grains and serve.

510
CALORIES

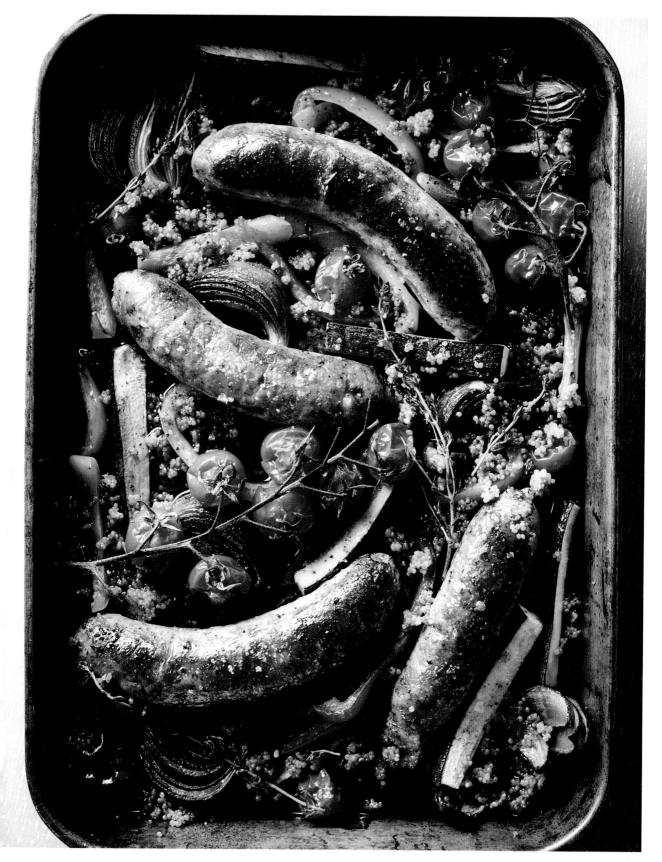

slow-cooking produces tender meat which is easy to digest. Anchovies add extra flavor and provide healthy fish oils.

Slow-Roasted Shoulder of Lamb

The meat portions here are generous but not huge as this is not a particularly high-protein diet. Evidence suggests that, while we need a minimum daily amount of protein (around 45-60g) because we are unable to store it, eating significantly more is not necessarily better, unless you are exercising a great deal.

Serves 8

3 garlic cloves, crushed

3 anchovies, chopped

2 tbsp olive oil

Juice of 1 large lemon

3 sprigs rosemary, leaves of
 1 sprig chopped

2½-3 lb shoulder of lamb

2 red onions, peeled
 and halved

8 oz red wine

•DAIRY-FREE

•GLUTEN-FREE

•GOOD FOR PHASE 1

1. Make a marinade by mixing together the garlic, anchovies, oil, lemon juice, and chopped rosemary leaves. Slash the surface of the meat in several places and place it in a nonmetallic dish. Rub in the marinade. Refrigerate the lamb to absorb the flavors and soften, 2-3 hours or overnight.

2. Take the lamb out of the fridge 30 minutes before cooking to bring it up to room temperature. Preheat the oven to 285°F.

3. Place the onions in a roasting pan and place the marinated meat on top. Pour any remaining marinade over the meat and tuck the 2 rosemary sprigs underneath. Pour the wine into the pan, along with ½ cup water. Cover the pan with a foil tent.

4. Roast the lamb for 4 hours, basting occasionally. Add water as needed if the juices start to dry out. Remove the foil for the last 20-30 minutes of cooking time, or once the meat is tender.

5. Serve the lamb with Cauliflower Baked with Lemon and Almonds (page 95), Roasted Purple Carrots with Tarragon (page 171), and greens of your choice (add 20 calories). There should be plenty of juices in the pan for gravy.

430 CALORIES

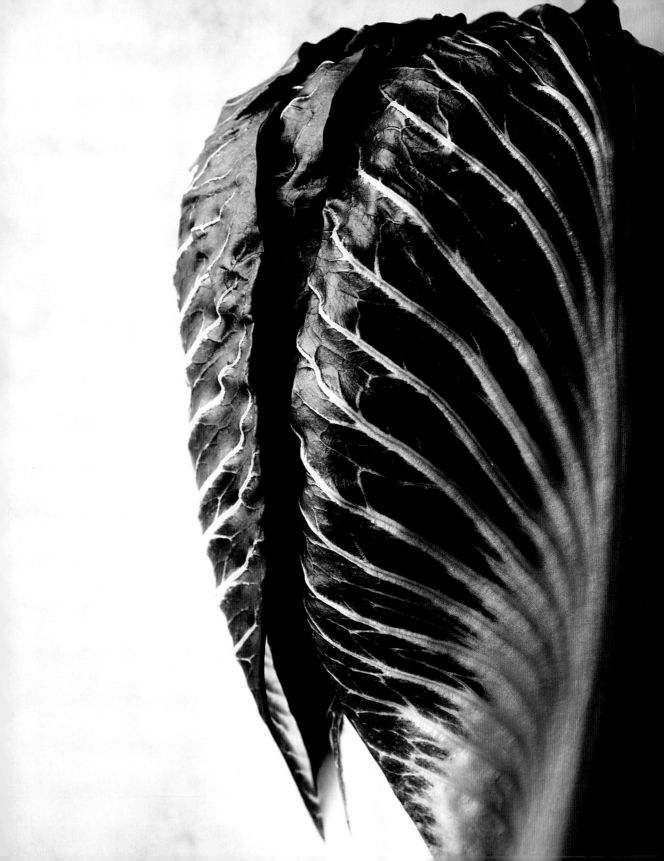

CLEVER VEGETABLES

Eating more vegetables is one
of the best ways of increasing the
diversity of your gut microbes,
and the greater the variety you
eat, the better. Whatever you are
cooking, consider adding one of
these dishes on the side.

Creamy Nutmeg Spinach

A great way to jazz up spinach.

Serves 2

1 pat butter, or 1 tbsp
   light olive oil
½ small onion, finely diced
1 garlic clove, crushed
½ tsp grated nutmeg
7 oz fresh spinach, tough
   stalks removed (or
   thawed frozen)
¼ cup crème fraîche
   (or soy cream)
⅓ cup grated Parmesan
   (or vegan Parmesan)

•DAIRY-FREE OPTION
•GLUTEN-FREE
•GOOD FOR PHASE 1

1. Heat the butter in a frying pan or wok. Sauté the onion gently over medium heat for 4-5 minutes, then add the garlic and nutmeg and cook for another 2 minutes.

2. Add the spinach and cook, stirring occasionally, until it starts to wilt. Stir in the crème fraîche and Parmesan and let it simmer for a couple of minutes. Serve piping hot.

240 CALORIES

Scorched Purple Radicchio

Charring the radicchio adds a wonderful caramelized, lightly smoked flavor to the leaves. The more bitter the leaves, the better they tend to be for both you and your microbiome.

Serves 2

½ head radicchio, cut in half
Squeeze of lemon juice

•DAIRY-FREE
•GLUTEN-FREE
•GOOD FOR PHASE 1

1. Preheat the broiler. Place the radicchio on a baking sheet, cut side up, and season with salt and pepper. Broil until the edges are starting to char, about 3 minutes.

2. Squeeze some lemon on top and serve.

Tip: The radicchio can also be cooked on a grill pan or outdoor grill for enhanced smokiness.

10 CALORIES

Quick Garlic-Fried Greens

Do as the Mediterraneans do. Simple.

Serves 2

5 oz dark leafy greens, such as mature spinach, spring greens, Swiss chard, or kale, chopped and tough stalks removed

2 tbsp olive oil

1 garlic clove, finely chopped

Grated zest of ½ lemon, plus a small squeeze of juice

¼ cup grated Parmesan or pecorino cheese (or vegan Parmesan)

•DAIRY-FREE OPTION

•GLUTEN-FREE

•GOOD FOR PHASE 1

1. Steam or boil the greens until they are just starting to soften, then drain.

2. Heat the oil in a frying pan over medium heat and add the garlic, followed by the greens. Sprinkle the lemon zest and Parmesan on top and cook for a couple of minutes. Season with freshly ground black pepper and a squeeze of lemon.

Note: For most people, the "scratchy," tough fiber in the stalks of cabbage or kale, or the stringy bits in beans, is well tolerated, particularly if chewed properly. But those with IBS may need to reduce the amount they eat and go easy with beans and lentils, too, as these can exacerbate bloating and cramps. (For more on FODMAPS in IBS see page 24).

290 CALORIES

Pea and Edamame Mash

Peas and edamame beans provide fiber, protein, and other vital nutrients.

Serves 2

⅔ cup frozen shelled
  edamame
¾ cup frozen baby peas
2 tbsp full-fat active
  Greek-style yogurt
  (or soy cream)
2-3 mint leaves, chopped
Juice of 1 lime

•DAIRY-FREE OPTION
•GLUTEN-FREE
•GOOD FOR PHASE 1

1. Bring a pan of salted water to a boil, and cook the edamame for 2-3 minutes. Add the peas and cook for 5 minutes. Drain and transfer to a bowl. Mix in the yogurt, mint, and lime juice. Season with salt and black pepper.

2. Using a potato masher, coarsely mash most of the peas and beans until you have the consistency you like. For a smoother consistency, use a hand blender.

Note: If you have IBS, you might want to reduce your portion size.

150 CALORIES

Onion and Zucchini Bhajis

These bhajis—spicy Indian fritters—have been a huge hit in our household. Mixing turmeric with black pepper boosts its anti-inflammatory effect.

Serves 4

⅔ cup chickpea flour
  (besan)
½ tsp ground coriander
½ tsp cumin seeds
1 tsp ground turmeric
1 medium onion, thinly
  sliced
½ medium zucchini,
  grated
1 egg, beaten
3 tbsp rapeseed oil or ghee

•DAIRY-FREE OPTION
•GLUTEN-FREE
•GOOD FOR PHASE 1

1. Mix the flour, coriander, cumin, and turmeric in a bowl and season with salt and black pepper. Add the onion and zucchini and stir until well combined, then stir in the egg.

2. Heat the oil in a frying pan over medium heat. Drop heaped tablespoonfuls of the mixture into the pan, flattening them slightly. Fry for 1-2 minutes per side, until crisp and golden brown. Remove from the pan with a slotted spoon and place on paper towels to drain.

Note: Onions are good for your microbiome, but these may be too much of a good thing if you have IBS.

190 CALORIES

Green Banana and Pepper Stir-Fry

This is a great side dish with lots of crunch and a slightly fruity flavor. When gently fried, unripe bananas taste more like sweet potatoes; they are more gut-friendly than potatoes, however, as the starch they contain is resistant, i.e., not rapidly converted to sugar.

Serves 4

3 tbsp olive oil
1 red onion, sliced
1 red bell pepper, seeded
   and chopped
1 yellow bell pepper,
   seeded and chopped
1 tsp cumin seeds
2 green bananas, sliced
Handful of fresh cilantro
   leaves, torn

• DAIRY-FREE
• GLUTEN-FREE
• OPTION FOR PHASE 1

1. Heat the oil in a wok or large frying pan and sauté the onion for 2 minutes.

2. Add the bell peppers and cumin seeds and stir-fry for 8-10 minutes, until the bell peppers start to soften slightly and the onion starts to caramelize.

3. Add the banana slices and cook for 3-4 minutes, or until golden brown.

4. Before serving, sprinkle the cilantro and some freshly ground black pepper on top.

Note: Green bananas are not ideal for IBS sufferers due to the "scratchy" fiber they contain. For Phase 1 we suggest reducing the onion by half and replacing 1 of the bell peppers with 5 oz broccoli.

170 CALORIES

Smoky Eggplant and Cannellini Beans

Based on the Middle Eastern dish baba ghanoush, this makes a wonderful side dish or dip. Those with IBS, or in the first two weeks of Phase 1, may find the fiber in it exacerbates symptoms, in which case reduce your portion size or swap out the beans for chickpeas.

Serves 4 as a side dish

1 medium eggplant
(about 8 oz)

5 tbsp olive oil

1 onion, diced

2 large garlic cloves,
crushed

2 tsp chopped fresh herbs,
such as thyme, parsley, or
oregano (or 1 tsp dried)

½ cup canned white beans
such as cannellini
or chickpeas, rinsed and
drained

1 tbsp balsamic vinegar

½ tsp red pepper flakes
(optional)

Handful of fresh
cilantro, chopped

•DAIRY-FREE
•GLUTEN-FREE

1. To give the eggplant the distinctive smoky flavor, roast it whole, stalk still attached, in a wok or saucepan with the lid on over high heat. Allow the skin to char in places before turning it. Aim to char more than half the skin—this will take 4-5 minutes. Place on a plate and allow the eggplant to cool. For alternative charring techniques, see tip below.

2. Using a knife, remove the stalk, then peel and discard the skin. Dice the flesh, retaining any browned parts as these add to the flavor.

3. Heat the oil in a medium saucepan and sauté the onion for about 5 minutes without letting it brown. Add the garlic, herbs, eggplant, and beans. Mix in the vinegar and red pepper flakes to taste. Add 2-3 tbsp water to loosen the mixture.

4. Cover the pan and simmer for 12-15 minutes, stirring occasionally. Add 1-2 tbsp water at a time if it is drying out, to maintain a thick, creamy texture. Season with salt and freshly ground black pepper and stir in half the cilantro. Before serving, scatter the remaining cilantro on top. For a creamier texture, or if you wish to serve it as a dip, blitz the mixture briefly with a hand blender.

Tip: Another way to char the eggplant is to hold it directly over a hot flame on the stovetop. Or pierce it and place it under the broiler, turning it so it chars evenly. Then remove the skin as described above.

220 CALORIES

Eggplant is an excellent source of fiber and vitamins B1 and B6, as well as minerals such as potassium, copper, magnesium, and manganese. It is also rich in antioxidants, specifically nasunin, which is found in the dark purple skin.

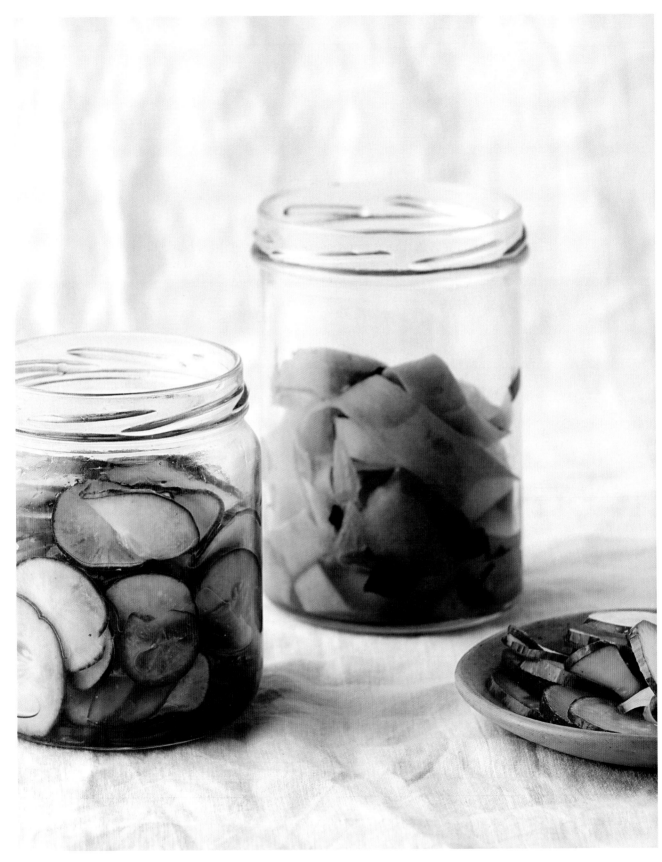

Japanese-Style Quick-Pickled Vegetables

Thinly sliced vegetables that have been lightly pickled add a delicate Japanese flavor to many dishes. Great with fish or seafood.

Serves 2

¼ cucumber

3 radishes

Generous pinch of Maldon
  sea salt

1 tsp raw unfiltered organic
  apple cider vinegar

1 tsp mirin wine (optional)

•DAIRY-FREE

•GLUTEN-FREE

•GOOD FOR PHASE 1

1. Slice the cucumber and radishes thinly, ideally with a mandoline, then place in a small dish, with the salt, vinegar, and mirin.

2. Using your fingers, massage in the salt and then leave the vegetables to rest for about 20 minutes. Store in the fridge for up to 2 days.

Tips: Use a Y-shaped slicer or mandoline to cut longer slices of carrot or zucchini to add to the dish. For extra flavor add strips of dried nori seaweed.

20 CALORIES

Vegetable-Rich Tomato Sauce

A rich and versatile tomato sauce full of hidden goodness. Even determined vegetable avoiders are likely to enjoy it. This will keep in the fridge for up to five days or in the freezer for up to two months. Keep portions in the freezer ready to use.

Makes about 5 cups,
or 4 servings

½ cup olive oil

1 large onion, diced

2 garlic cloves, diced

2 celery stalks, diced

2 carrots, diced

2 medium zucchini, diced

2 red bell peppers, seeded
and diced

1 tbsp chopped fresh
oregano or basil, or 1 tsp
dried oregano

1 large bay leaf

½ tsp dried thyme

2 (14-oz) cans diced
tomatoes

1 (15-oz) can pumpkin
puree

2 tbsp balsamic vinegar

•DAIRY-FREE

•GLUTEN-FREE

•GOOD FOR PHASE 1

1. Heat the oil in a large saucepan over medium heat. Add the onion, garlic, celery, carrots, zucchini, and bell peppers and sweat for 10-15 minutes, stirring frequently. In the last few minutes add the herbs.

2. Add the tomatoes, pumpkin puree, vinegar, and 1¼ cups water and cover. Simmer for at least 30 minutes—ideally for up to an hour. You may need to add extra water if it is getting too thick, or remove the lid if it needs thickening.

3. Discard the bay leaf. When the vegetables are soft and the sauce is the desired consistency, blitz it briefly with a hand blender, leaving some chunky bits for texture. Season to taste.

Tips: You can use this tomato sauce in a variety of ways, for example as a base for meat or fish dishes, or to pour over vegetables or pasta. Change the selection of herbs to get different flavors. It also works well as a base for soup (see Spicy Lentil and Tomato Soup, page 62).

370
CALORIES

Puy Lentils with Balsamic Vinegar

With their uniquely peppery flavor and ability to keep their shape and texture when cooked, Puy lentils are a cut above other lentils, containing plenty of fiber and some protein, too. Delicious served hot or cold.

Serves 4
(2-4 as a side dish)

¼ cup olive oil

1 onion, diced

1 celery stalk, diced

1 garlic clove, finely
  chopped

8 oz Puy lentils

2 tbsp balsamic vinegar

1 tsp fresh thyme, or ½ tsp
  dried

2 cups vegetable stock
  (or water)

Handful of fresh cilantro,
  chopped

•DAIRY-FREE
•GLUTEN-FREE

1. Heat the oil in a medium saucepan and sauté the onion and celery over medium heat for 4-5 minutes, stirring occasionally. They should be soft but not browned.

2. Add the garlic and lentils and cook for another minute or so, then stir in the vinegar, thyme, and stock (or water). Add water, if needed, to cover the lentils by ½ inch.

3. Bring to a boil and simmer, covered, for 20-25 minutes, until the lentils are firm to the bite. Season with salt and pepper and stir in the cilantro before serving.

Tip: Serve on a bed of salad leaves with a sprinkling of crumbled feta and sliced avocado for a light meal.

Note: The fiber in lentils can make IBS worse. Reduce your portion size, or avoid them altogether in Phase 1.

240 CALORIES

Roasted Vegetables

There is something wonderfully comforting about a pan of steaming, caramelized vegetables straight from the oven. Roasted vegetables also have more flavor and tend to be easier to digest.

Beets Roasted in Their Skins

Probably our favorite way of cooking beets, one which leaves all the goodness intact as most of the nutrients reside in the skin. They make a great accompaniment to lots of dishes.

Serves 2

6 oz small beets, scrubbed, trimmed, and cut into quarters

2 tbsp olive oil

½ tsp cumin seeds

Pinch of red pepper flakes, or to taste

1 tbsp raw unfiltered apple cider vinegar

• DAIRY-FREE
• GLUTEN-FREE
• GOOD FOR PHASE 1

1. Preheat the oven to 350°F. Place the beets in a roasting pan, then toss them with the oil, cumin seeds, red pepper flakes, sea salt, and freshly ground black pepper.

2. Cover the pan with foil and bake for 20 minutes. Remove the foil, drizzle over the vinegar and return to the oven. Bake, uncovered, for 15-20 minutes longer, or until the beets are tender and starting to brown.

3. Serve with bitter greens such as arugula, dandelion greens, or baby spinach (add 10 calories).

Tip: For a more substantial meal, add smoked fish, cold meats, or some cheese.

150 CALORIES

Roasted Jerusalem Artichokes

Artichokes are knobbly and tedious to peel—so much easier to just give them a good scrub (thus retaining the best of the nutrients in the skin). Baked in the oven, they come out sweet and tasty, with an earthy succulence, and are loaded with gut-friendly soluble fiber, as well as iron, potassium, and vitamin B_1.

Serves 4

1 lb Jerusalem artichokes, scrubbed, cut in half if large
2 tbsp olive oil
Juice of ½ lemon

•DAIRY-FREE
•GLUTEN-FREE

1. Preheat the oven to 350°F. Place the artichokes in a baking dish, toss with the oil, and season with salt and pepper.

2. Roast the artichokes for about 45 minutes, or until tender. Drizzle with the lemon juice before serving.

260 CALORIES

Roasted Purple Carrots with Tarragon

Cooking carrots, particularly with their skin still on, helps to increase the absorption of nutrients such as beta-carotene; adding plenty of olive oil enhances the absorption of fat-soluble vitamins.

Serves 2

8 oz purple (or orange) carrots, scrubbed and trimmed
3 tbsp extra-virgin olive oil
1 tsp dried tarragon
Juice of ½ lemon

•DAIRY-FREE
•GLUTEN-FREE
•GOOD FOR PHASE 1

1. Preheat the oven to 350°F. Place the carrots in a baking dish or roasting pan. Toss with the oil, tarragon, and season with salt and pepper.

2. Bake for 20-30 minutes, stirring occasionally, until they start to brown. Drizzle with the lemon juice before serving.

Tip: Delicious served with Slow-Roasted Shoulder of Lamb (page 157) or Beef and Orange Stew with Mushrooms (page 150).

220 CALORIES

Roasted Butternut Squash

A simple, gut-friendly side dish, which boosts fiber intake and is generally very well tolerated.

Serves 2
½ small butternut squash, peeled
3 tbsp olive oil
1 tbsp grated Parmesan (or vegan Parmesan)
Juice of ½ lemon

•DAIRY-FREE OPTION
•GLUTEN-FREE
•GOOD FOR PHASE 1

1. Preheat the oven to 350°F. Slice the butternut squash in half lengthwise. Scoop out the seeds and stringy bits and cut the flesh into long slices or semicircles.

2. Spread the slices in a baking dish and toss with the oil and season with salt and black pepper. Bake for 25-30 minutes, turning occasionally, until they start to brown and feel tender when pierced. Sprinkle the Parmesan over and bake for 5-6 minutes longer. Drizzle with the lemon juice before serving.

240 CALORIES

Slow-Roasted Tomatoes

Wonderful with Simple Creamy Scrambled Eggs (page 37) for breakfast, or added to a salad.

Serves 2
4 medium vine-ripened tomatoes, cut in half around the middle
2 tbsp olive oil
1 garlic clove, minced
2 tsp fresh herbs, such as thyme or rosemary, leaves only (or 1 tsp dried)

•DAIRY-FREE
•GLUTEN-FREE
•GOOD FOR PHASE 1

1. Preheat the oven to 250°F.

2. Place the tomatoes cut side up in a baking dish. Drizzle with the oil and scatter the garlic and herbs on top. Season well with salt and black pepper.

3. Bake for 3½-4 hours, until the tomatoes are soft and caramelized.

170 CALORIES

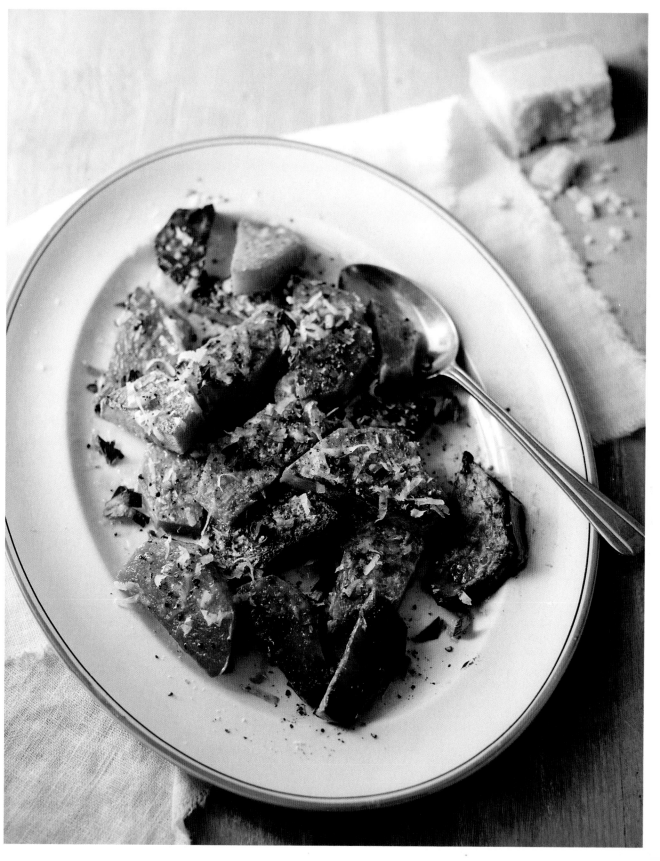

Healthy Swaps

You will have gathered by now that your gut does not thrive on foods that are sweet or starchy. Nor do they help your blood sugar or waistline, let alone your metabolism. Try some of these alternatives to potatoes, rice, pasta, and noodles. There are suggestions for healthy breads in the Treats chapter, too.

Cauliflower Rice with Cilantro

An ideal low-carb, gut-friendly alternative to rice to mop up the juices of a curry or stew. Cauliflower contains some of almost every mineral and vitamin you need. And to top it all, it's high in fiber and antioxidants. Amazing that so much can be packed into such a pale and unassuming vegetable.

Serves 4
2 tbsp olive oil
1 small onion, finely
  chopped
1 small garlic clove,
  finely chopped (optional)
1 medium cauliflower
Large handful of fresh
  cilantro, chopped

•DAIRY-FREE
•GLUTEN-FREE
•GOOD FOR PHASE 1

1. Heat the oil in a pan and sauté the onion and garlic for 4-5 minutes.

2. Meanwhile, chop the cauliflower into florets and grate it or use a food processor to turn it into "rice." It should look a bit like pale bulgur wheat.

3. Add the cauliflower rice to the pan, then turn up the heat, and stir-fry until it is al dente, 6-7 minutes. Add the cilantro, season with salt and pepper, and serve.

70 CALORIES

Eggplant Chips

These make a crisp, tasty, and healthy alternative to starchy, sugar-spiking potato chips. Great with a light salad or to eat with a dip.

Serves 4

1 cup ground almonds

½ tsp cayenne pepper

1 egg

1 medium eggplant, cut into thin slices

3 tbsp light olive oil

•DAIRY-FREE

•GLUTEN-FREE

•GOOD FOR PHASE 1

1. Preheat the oven to 400°F. Mix the almonds and cayenne on a plate. Beat the egg in a bowl.

2. Dip each eggplant slice first into the egg and then into the almond mixture. Repeat to ensure the chips get a good even coating. Season generously with salt and freshly ground black pepper.

3. Place the chips on a greased baking sheet and drizzle over the oil. Bake for 15-20 minutes, or until golden brown. Serve with Avocado and Lime Salsa (page 75) or one of our delicious dips (pages 72-74).

280 CALORIES

Red Rice with Resistant Starch

Red rice has the same relatively low GI as brown rice but contains extra nutrients, such as healthy polyphenols. The process of cooking then cooling the rice in the fridge for 12 hours converts some of the starchy carbohydrates into resistant starch. This gut-friendly form of fiber is not absorbed in the small intestine, but instead makes its way to the large bowel and feeds your "good" bacteria.

Serves 4

½ cup red Camargue rice

½ cup brown rice

1 tsp coconut oil or mild olive oil

•DAIRY-FREE

•GLUTEN-FREE

•GOOD FOR PHASE 1

1. Place the rice in a saucepan with a lid. Cover with twice its volume of water and add the oil and a pinch of salt. Bring to a boil, cover, and simmer for 20-30 minutes, or until most of the water has been absorbed. Turn the heat off and leave the pot covered to steam the rice for another 5-10 minutes.

2. Allow the rice to cool before putting it in the fridge for 12 hours/overnight to convert more of the starch into gut-friendly resistant starch.

3. The rice is then ready to use, either cold or reheated—for example in a rice salad (page 90) or as a rice pudding (page 213). You also get the same benefit if you freeze it in portions.

Tip: You can use either red or brown rice on its own for this recipe; using both just adds a bit more texture and flavor.

90 CALORIES

Pan-Fried Zucchini Spaghetti

These days we often swap starchy spaghetti for "noodles" made from fresh, firm vegetables such as squash or carrot. You can also go for a half-and-half version: Boil a small portion of spaghetti and throw spiralized zucchini into the pot for the last minute of cooking. Once you get a taste for it you will probably find you'll want to abandon the spaghetti altogether.

Serves 2

2 tbsp olive oil

2 large zucchini, spiralized

1 small garlic clove, crushed (optional)

Squeeze of lemon

•DAIRY-FREE

•GLUTEN-FREE

•GOOD FOR PHASE 1

1. Heat a large frying pan over medium heat. Add the oil and fry the zucchini with the garlic for 1-1½ minutes, stirring frequently. It needs to remain al dente, so don't overcook or it will become soggy.

2. Season with Maldon sea salt, freshly ground black pepper, and a squeeze of lemon, and serve immediately with a main dish, such as Turkey and Mushroom Bolognese (page 131) or Vegetable-Rich Tomato Sauce (page 168).

130 CALORIES

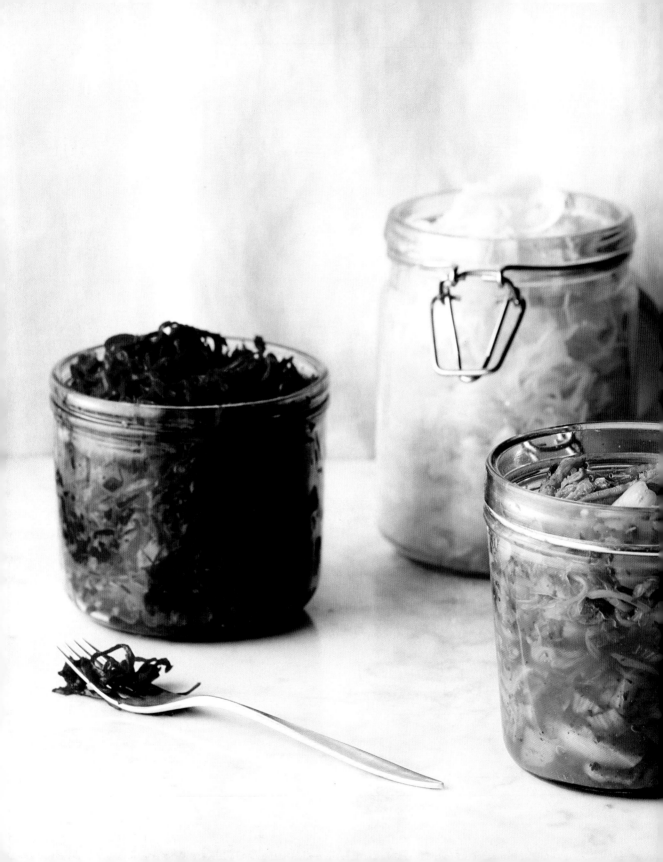

FERMENTS

Fermenting is making a comeback in
kitchens around the world—and for
good reason. It's cheap, it's fun, and
there is hardly a better way of nurturing
the good guys in your gut. We should
all have some jars of interesting things
fizzing away on the counter.

Kombucha

Kombucha is a fermented tea that has been brewed for millennia in China, Russia, and Eastern Europe. It makes a refreshing drink with a subtle apple flavor and a sweet-and-sour fizz. It is produced by a living organism, or "mother," known as a symbiotic culture of bacteria and yeast (or SCOBY), a complex culture of microorganisms that acts as a probiotic, providing your gut with healthy microbes.

Kombucha is an easy and forgiving ferment to manage. First you need to source your SCOBY—you can buy them online (see cleverguts.com). It looks somewhat like a squashed beige jellyfish and floats like a rubbery raft on or in the tea, protecting and maintaining the fermentation. To encourage the aerobic process, the brew needs to be open to fresh air. The recipe below is for a relatively low-sugar version. Calorie counts are not included as much of the sugar added is used up in the fermentation process. How much remains depends on how many days you ferment it.

Makes 1 quart

1 SCOBY

1 quart spring or filtered water (tap water contains chlorine which can prevent fermentation)

2-3 tea bags, ideally organic black, green, or white tea (your kombucha will probably prefer some teas to others as each SCOBY is unique; see page 182)

⅓ cup unbleached sugar

You will also need:

2 (1-quart) wide-mouth glass jars

1 (1-quart) glass bottle with tight-fitting lid

Small piece of cloth or muslin

•DAIRY-FREE

•GLUTEN-FREE

1. Place your SCOBY, along with its fluid, in one jar and set aside.

2. Bring about 1¼ cups of the filtered water to a boil. Add to the second jar, along with the tea bags and sugar, and let steep for 30 minutes. Remove the tea bags and pour in the remaining water to make almost 1 quart of sweetened tea. Let cool.

3. Once the tea is at room temperature you can add it to the jar with the SCOBY. If it is too hot it will kill the SCOBY. The water level in the jar needs to remain at least ¾ inch below the top of the jar. Cover it with a clean piece of moderately tightly woven cloth, to keep out dust and bugs yet still allow airflow. (Muslin is not quite densely woven enough, though you could use 2 or 3 layers of it.) Secure the cloth with a rubber band. Don't use a lid as it needs the air. Then leave it to brew on the kitchen counter out of direct sunlight at room temperature.

4. After a few days you will notice small bubbles forming around the edge of the SCOBY. Your alien life-form is springing into action! If you lift the cloth you will notice a delicious sweet, slightly tart smell. Pale brownish stringy floaty bits will probably accumulate below the SCOBY and the liquid may become a bit cloudy. That's fine.

5. It will be ready to drink after around 5 days but can be brewed for longer according to taste, as it develops a richer, tarter flavor with a slight fizz. Use a clean spoon to taste a little. It is probably best decanted within 2 weeks. The longer it is left, the more vinegary and fizzy it becomes.

6. When it's ready, decant the liquid into a clean glass bottle with a tight lid. Leave behind roughly the same volume of fluid as the size of the SCOBY, so it can be restarted in the next few days by adding more sweetened tea to repeat the cycle. Place the bottle in the fridge, leaving only about ½ inch air under the lid, to halt the aerobic process and prevent further fermenting. This also helps to stop it turning to vinegar (though you can use that in cooking). As it is a live ferment, the container might burst or leak if it is left in a warm place.

Tips: Though kombucha is usually well tolerated, we suggest starting with a small glass so you can introduce it to your gut gradually. Some people prefer to drink it diluted with water.

Only use black or green tea that has come from the tea plant *Camellia*
sinensis. Herbal infusions are not technically tea; they are simply herbs or fruits
infused in boiling water (this includes rooibos tea). When we added a peppermint
tea bag to a second brew, the SCOBY went moldy and had to be discarded. Some
cultures thrive better on one type of tea than another, depending on what it was
originally grown in. So, if you have a spare SCOBY, experiment and see what works
for yours. Green tea is a particularly popular flavor and may have extra health
benefits, too.

Don't store the SCOBY in the fridge. It may survive for short periods, but the
cold will weaken it and it may take time to recover, or not recover at all. You should
of course store the bottled kombucha in the fridge.

It is not thriving if you see patches of black mold or if it smells unpleasant,
rancid, or "cheesy." If this happens, sadly you will need to discard it and start again.

If you are away for a few weeks, simply make a fresh batch and leave it to do its
own thing. You may find that it has turned to vinegar on your return, but the SCOBY
will be fine. Decant most of the fluid as usual, then top it off again with fresh sweet tea.

Managing the SCOBY: Over a matter of weeks the SCOBY will gradually get
thicker, more uniform in shape, and float on top. When it has grown to about a ½-inch
thickness you can split it to make 2 thinner disks or cut a chunk off it. Remove the
extra disk and place it in a jar along with at least twice its volume in fluid from the
"mother." This can be kept as a spare, just in case, or to pass on to other "boochas"
to grow their own.

Storing kombucha: When a spare kombucha has been allowed to rest, you need
to add about ¼ cup sugar every 4-6 weeks to keep it alive. Then every 2-3 months,
discard most of the liquid in your kombucha "hotel" and top off the jar to four-fifths
with fresh sweet tea to keep it going.

Kombucha is thought to confer beneficial health effects through its high levels of polyphenols and other antioxidants. Recent studies have also revealed evidence of possible anti-cancer properties.

Preserved Lemons

Lemon peel contains twice the amount of vitamins as lemon flesh, and has a more intense flavor than the juice, with a hint of bitterness. Once fermented, the flavors mellow and the peel softens. Preserved lemon works wonderfully in small quantities in both sweet and savory dishes such as Easy Chicken Tagine (page 127), Lemony Buttermilk Dressing (page 118), and Cauliflower Baked with Lemon and Almonds (page 95). The majority of store-bought preserved lemons are devoid of live bacteria, and in our experience can have an industrial mouthwash taste to them. So it is well worth making your own.

Makes 1 cup

6-7 large unwaxed
    lemons, preferably organic
1 tbsp raw unfiltered apple
    cider vinegar
1 heaping tbsp Maldon
    sea salt
½ tsp coriander seeds
    (optional)

You will also need:
8-oz glass jar with
    well-fitting lid

•DAIRY-FREE
•GLUTEN-FREE
•GOOD FOR PHASE 1

1. Wash the lemons. Cut them in half and squeeze some of the juice from each into the jar. Then cut the halves in half again. Slice each lemon quarter finely, discarding the seeds and some of the pith.

2. Add the vinegar, then pack the slices tightly into the jar, scattering a generous pinch of salt and coriander seeds between the layers until the salt is used up.

3. Use a wooden spoon or the end of a rolling pin to squash the lemon slices down and force out the air bubbles. There should be enough juice to cover them. If necessary, add salted filtered or spring water, using 1 heaping tsp sea salt to ¾ cup water. As it's an anaerobic process, prevent contact with the air by covering the surface with a small dish, or adding a clean stone or ceramic or glass object to the liquid to raise it above the lemons before closing the jar.

4. For the first few days you need to "burp" the lemons a couple of times a day to release any trapped bubbles produced by fermentation. This means pressing them down so that they are always submerged. Leave them to ferment at room temperature for 5 days to 2 weeks. Then store them in the fridge to prevent further fermentation.

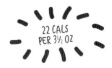
22 CALS
PER 3½ OZ

Red Cabbage Sauerkraut

This crunchy, dark red sauerkraut is one of our favorites. As well as the wonderful burst of color it brings to a meal, it has an appealing sweet-and-sour flavor. What's more, it's packed with those healthy phytonutrients found in colored vegetables. It can be served with almost any food, including for breakfast.

Makes 1 quart

4 tsp Maldon sea salt

1 small red cabbage (about 2 lb), core and outer leaves removed, chopped

2 medium onions, chopped

1 tsp mustard seeds

1 tsp coriander seeds, toasted

½-1 tsp red pepper flakes

You will also need:

1-quart glass jar with well-fitting lid

•DAIRY-FREE

•GLUTEN-FREE

1. In a large bowl, massage the salt into the cabbage and onion, mixing in the mustard seeds, coriander seeds, and red pepper flakes at the same time. Leave them to sweat for 1-2 hours. The liquid from the vegetables will collect in the bottom of the bowl. Reserve it for later.

2. Transfer the salted vegetables to the jar, cramming them in with clean hands or the end of a wooden rolling pin. Pour in the reserved liquid from the bowl and push the vegetables firmly down again. The liquid should rise above the surface.

3. If there is not enough liquid, even after a few hours, you can top it off with brine made with 1 tsp Maldon sea salt dissolved in ¾ cup filtered water. The water level should be about ½ inch above the vegetables and about 1 inch below the top of the jar. Place a clean stone, ceramic, or glass object on top of the vegetables to raise the liquid and keep them submerged.

4. Leave the sauerkraut to stand on the counter out of direct sunlight for 3-14 days, depending on the room temperature and how the taste is developing. Test it regularly for flavor. Then store in a sealed jar in the fridge. It will keep for a few months.

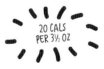

20 CALS PER 3½ OZ

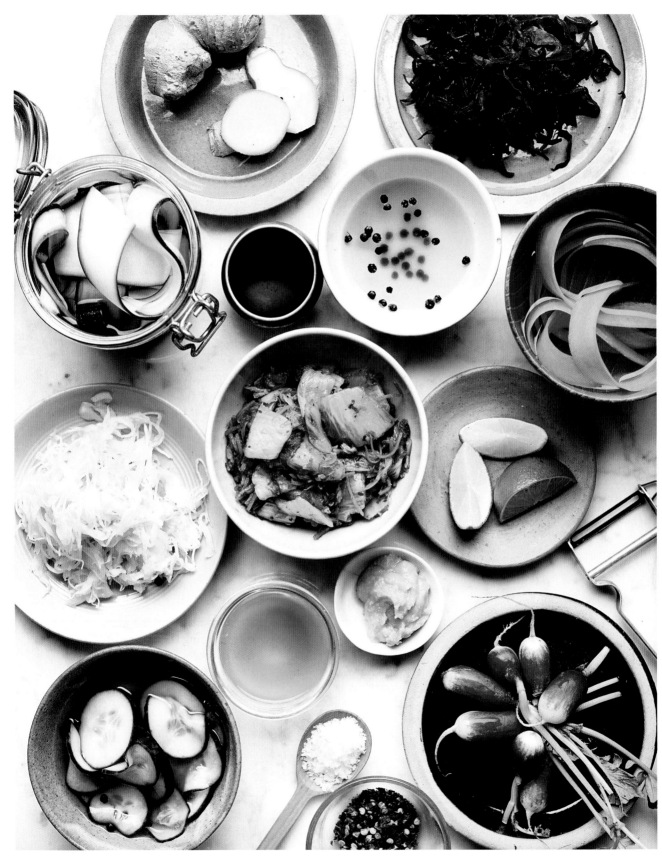

Fermented Pickled Vegetables

Once you get going, the principles of fermentation are simple and you can start working with all sorts of different vegetables.

Makes 1 quart

2 lb tough vegetables, such as cabbage, beets, onions, radishes, or carrots, or a mixture of all, thinly sliced

4-5 tsp Maldon sea salt

Flavoring, such as 1 tsp mustard seeds, fennel seeds, coriander seeds, red pepper flakes, or peppercorns; and herbs, such as a small bunch of dill, a sprig of rosemary, or 1-2 bay leaves

You will also need:

1-quart glass jar with well-fitting lid

•DAIRY-FREE
•GLUTEN-FREE

Massage and press all the ingredients together in a large bowl, scattering salt over as you go. Then transfer them to the jar and press them down firmly with the end of a rolling pin or wooden spoon, leaving 1-inch headspace. Let them rest for 30-60 minutes, to allow the salt to draw the liquid out of them.

The vegetables need to be kept submerged, as it is an anaerobic process. Place a heavy object on the surface, such as a glass dish, to prevent contact with the air. If there isn't enough liquid to cover the vegetables, make extra brine by dissolving 1 tsp salt in ¾ cup filtered water. (Tap water contains chlorine which kills bacteria.) Seal the jar tightly. Leave it at room temperature, away from direct sunlight.

For the first 3-4 days the vegetables need to be "burped" a couple of times a day, to release the gases that are a by-product of fermentation. Press down on the vegetables using a wooden spoon or the end of a rolling pin to release trapped bubbles. Taste the vegetables occasionally. They gradually get sweeter and softer. When they are ready—soft with a bit of crunch (after 5-14 days)—place the sealed jar in the fridge to prevent further fermentation. The vegetables will keep for a few months.

You can vary the fermentation by changing the kind of vegetable (or fruit) used, or by altering the saltiness. By adding different seasonings and seeds, you can also change the flavors. Be creative and try different combinations.

Pickled Zucchini with Mustard Seeds

Pickling is a traditional way of preserving vegetables and fruit at a time of plenty. Sadly, the word is now associated with sterile items that you pull off the supermarket shelves, almost certainly containing few live micro-organisms. This pickle goes with most meals—try it with Black Bean Beet Burgers (page 147) or fish. Or simply nibble on it before a meal to get those digestive juices flowing.

Makes 2 cups

10 oz mini zucchini,
    trimmed and sliced
    in half lengthwise
½ small white onion, sliced
2 tsp Maldon sea salt, plus
    ½ tbsp for the brine
1 tsp mustard seeds
1 tsp coriander seeds
½ tsp red pepper flakes
Small pinch of black tea
    leaves

You will also need:
16-oz glass jar with well-
    fitting lid

•DAIRY-FREE
•GLUTEN-FREE

30 CALS
PER 3½ OZ

1. Wash the zucchini under the tap and rinse them with filtered water to remove any remaining chlorine. Place them on a large plate cut side up and scatter the onion on top, followed by the 2 tsp salt. Leave them for 1-2 hours, until the salt has drawn the water out.

2. Toast the mustard and coriander seeds in a hot pan for a minute or two, to bring out the flavor. Put them in the jar, along with the red pepper flakes and the tea (the tannin in the tea helps the vegetables remain firm).

3. Add the vegetables to the jar, along with their liquid and any salt left on the plate. Tilt the jar slightly so the zucchini are packed standing upright.

4. Dissolve ½ tbsp salt in 1 cup filtered water. Pour this over the zucchini so that they're covered with about ½ inch liquid. Place a small glass or ceramic object on top to keep them submerged. If they dry out, top the jar off with brine made with 1 tsp salt to ¾ cup filtered water.

5. Stand the jar on the counter out of direct sunlight or excessive heat for 2-5 days. I prefer the vegetables after 2-3 days as they remain slightly more crunchy. Over the first 3 days or so, open the lid daily to release the fermentation gases. If it is active, you will see tiny bubbles forming as lactic acid ferments the sugars in the vegetables. When the pickles are ready, store in the fridge, where they will keep for 2-3 weeks.

Spicy Pickled Onions

Most pickled onion recipes seem to involve pouring boiling-hot vinegar and/or brine mixtures over the onions, which kills all the natural *Lactobacilli* and other microorganisms needed for fermentation and the production of probiotics. In this recipe, they are lightly pickled in microbiome-friendly cider vinegar. The result is a beautifully sweet, spicy pickle, which is great sliced and scattered on a salad, or nibbled with cheese.

Makes 1½ cups

½ tsp coriander seeds

½ tsp peppercorns

½ tsp mustard seeds

Pinch of red pepper flakes (optional)

About 12 oz shallots, or any small onions, peeled and trimmed

¾ cup raw unfiltered apple cider vinegar

You will also need:

12-oz glass jar with well-fitting lid

•DAIRY-FREE

•GLUTEN-FREE

1. Toast the coriander seeds in a hot pan for a minute or two to bring out the flavor, then put them in the jar with the other spices.

2. Cut the larger shallots or onions in half and add them to the jar until it is just over three-quarters full.

3. Dilute the vinegar by mixing it with ½ cup filtered water. Pour this into the jar—there should be about ½-inch liquid above the onions. Place a small glass or ceramic object on top to keep the onions submerged.

4. Leave them to ferment for 3-14 days. Taste regularly and, when you're happy with them, pop them in the fridge to prevent further fermentation. They will keep for 3-4 weeks. Drain or rinse off the vinegar before serving.

20 CALS PER 3½ OZ

Kefir Milk

Kefir is a fermented milk drink that tastes like a tangy, runny yogurt. The culture is grown either from powder or, more commonly, "grains," which look like tiny soft cauliflower florets. These contain a complex ecosystem of as many as 40-50 types of bacteria and yeasts, which work together to produce one of the most probiotic-rich drinks available.

Makes 1 quart
1 quart organic full-fat milk
Kefir starter powder
  or grains

You will also need:
1-quart glass container with
  lid (or cover with plastic
  wrap)

•GLUTEN-FREE

Kefir starter cultures: These are usually available as fresh grains or as dried powder in sachets. If you are lucky, you might be given fresh grains by a friend who has cultivated an excess. They can be reused repeatedly. Our kefir culture has been producing about a quart of kefir a week for some months now. You can also buy the cultures from health food stores or online (or go to cleverguts.com).

Kefir is best fermented between 72° and 75°F, over about 24 hours. It sets more quickly when warmer and can take up to 30 hours on a cold day. Avoid stirring it while it is fermenting.

If using fresh grains, add 2 tbsp for 2 cups organic full-fat milk. Drop them into the bottom of the jar and stir well. Leave it in a warm place.

If using powder, follow the instructions on the package, which are generally as follows: pour ½ cup of the milk into a container and mix with the powder to form a smooth paste. Then add the rest of the milk and stir for at least 5 minutes. (If you wish to produce more batches of kefir you can make up a bag of powder, a bit like a bouquet garni. To do this cut a circle of clean muslin about 4 inches in diameter and pour the powdered kefir into the center. Tie it into a bundle with a clean piece of string and place it in the bottom of the jar before adding the milk. Stir gently for 5 minutes to disperse some of the powder through the milk.)

The kefir milk is ready when it is lightly set.
At this point, scooping a spoonful out will leave a small indent in the surface. Once it has been stirred it looks like thin curdled milk. Strain all the contents through a fine sieve into a 1-quart jug. Use a spoon to gently scoop up the small grainy jellied lumps left in the sieve. Place the creamy kefir liquid in a covered glass jug or a bowl in the fridge to keep cool.

Keep the grains. These can be stored in a clean container in the fridge for a few days, just covered with kefir milk, until you are ready to add more milk and start the next batch of fermentation. If you get in the flow, after a month or two you will have more grains or a fuller muslin bag than you need. These can then be split, stored in the fridge, or given away to create another colony.

If using powder in a bundle, it should be discarded after a couple of months.

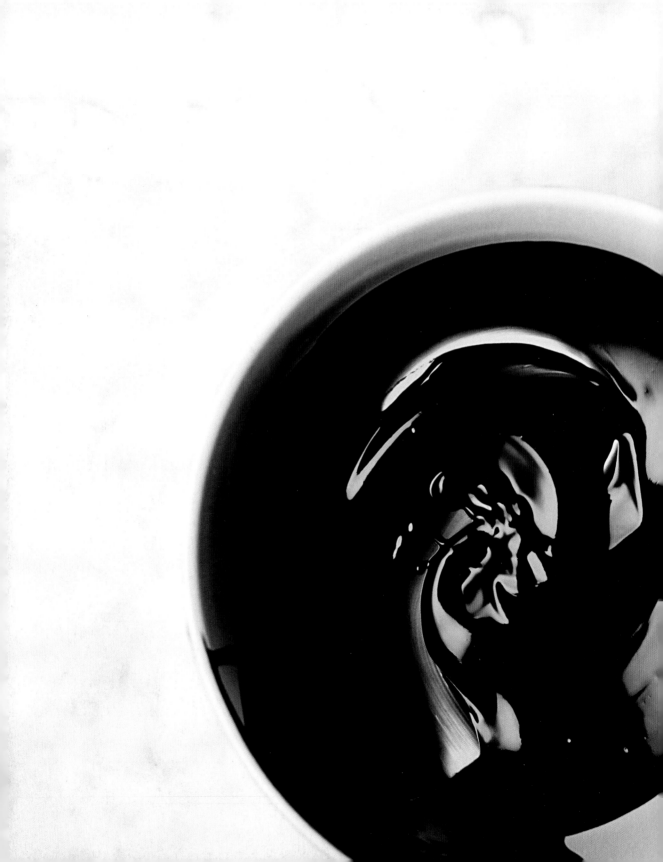

TREATS

Go for "good" treats that include a strong dose of healthy fiber and are relatively low in sugar. If you have a sweet tooth, it can take time to reset your taste buds. Stick with it—they will soon come back to life.

Breads

These breads are either gluten-free, or made with grains containing little gluten compared to that found in modern wheat. There is also a fermented sourdough, a traditional form of bread which the gut tolerates relatively well. Try them for breakfast with butter and scrambled eggs. Or enjoy them with Nut Butter (page 123), or a dollop of cream cheese and a spoonful of Strawberry Chia Jam (page 208). Just not too often!

Mug Bread

Instant, fresh, gluten-free, and delicious.

Makes 4 small round slices
2 tsp coconut oil
1 large egg
2 tbsp ground almonds or
    ground walnuts
3 tbsp ground flaxseeds
½ tsp baking powder
Generous pinch of salt

• DAIRY-FREE
• GLUTEN-FREE

1. Microwave the coconut oil in a mug with straight sides for 20-30 seconds on high, then use it to grease the sides of the mug.

2. In a small bowl, thoroughly mix together the egg, 2 tsp water, the almonds, flaxseeds, baking powder, and salt. Pour the mixture into the mug and stir with a fork to incorporate the coconut oil, making sure the top is level.

3. Microwave for 1 minute on high. If the bread still appears very moist, microwave for another 10-20 seconds. Avoid overcooking as this will make it rubbery.

4. Tip the bread out of the cup—it may need loosening with a knife. If it is still runny at the bottom, put it back in the cup and microwave it on high for another 10-20 seconds.

5. Allow it to cool for a few minutes on its side, then cut it into slices.

100 CALORIES PER SLICE

Whole Grain Flatbread

Flatbreads are easy to make and ideal for mopping up sauces, using in dips, or eating with salads. Unfortunately, store-bought white-flour flatbreads and chapatis tend to have a disastrous impact on blood sugar, driving weight gain and type 2 diabetes. This whole grain version will be absorbed more slowly and cause less of a blood sugar spike. The fiber will also nurture your good gut bacteria.

Makes 4
250g (2 cups plus 2 tbsp)
  whole grain flour,
  such as spelt (or use
  whole grain buckwheat or
  besan flour as a gluten-
  free option)
120ml (½ cup) cold water
40ml (2½ tbsp) olive oil
1 tsp baking powder
1 tsp salt and a grinding of
  black pepper

•DAIRY-FREE
•GLUTEN-FREE OPTION

1. Mix all the ingredients in a bowl to form a dough. Knead it briefly on a surface dusted with flour. Cover it and let it to rest for 30 minutes.

2. Divide the dough into 4 pieces and roll each into flat rounds approximately ⅓ inch thick on a lightly floured work surface. To prevent bubbles from forming, pierce each one a few times with a fork.

3. Heat a griddle or large frying pan and cook 1 flatbread at a time for 1-3 minutes. When it starts to brown, turn it over and cook it for 1-2 minutes on the other side. If a bubble appears, press it down gently to release the steam.

4. Serve the flatbreads warm, or cool them on a rack.

Note: Spelt is an ancient grain related to wheat but one which contains relatively lower amounts of gluten.

310 CALORIES

Seeded Soda Bread

A crispy loaf with added crunch and flavor thanks to the toasted seeds. This is another easy bread which doesn't require much kneading. The mildly acidic buttermilk or kefir reacts with the rising agent (baking soda) to produce carbon dioxide which creates the bubbles and does the leavening.

Makes 1 loaf
(about 10 slices)
200g (1⅔ cups) whole grain
   buckwheat flour
100g (¾ cup) all-purpose
   flour or gluten-free flour
1 tsp baking soda
35g (¼ cup) sunflower seeds
25g (¼ cup) sesame seeds
25g (3 tbsp) ground
   flaxseeds
25g (¼ cup) chia seeds
1 tbsp maple syrup
160ml (⅔ cup) kefir (see
   page 190) or buttermilk
A little milk for brushing

•GLUTEN-FREE OPTION

1. Preheat the oven to 400°F. In a bowl, mix the flours, baking soda, and two-thirds of the seeds. Make a well in the center and pour in the maple syrup and kefir and mix everything together to form a soft dough.

2. Turn the dough out onto a floured work surface and gently knead it. Make a round loaf and place it on a floured baking sheet. Cut a cross in the top with a sharp knife.

3. Brush the surface with a little milk, then sprinkle the remaining seeds over the top, pressing them in slightly. Bake the loaf for 30-35 minutes, until it sounds hollow when tapped underneath. Leave it to cool on a wire rack. It can be frozen on the day of baking.

190 CALORIES PER SLICE

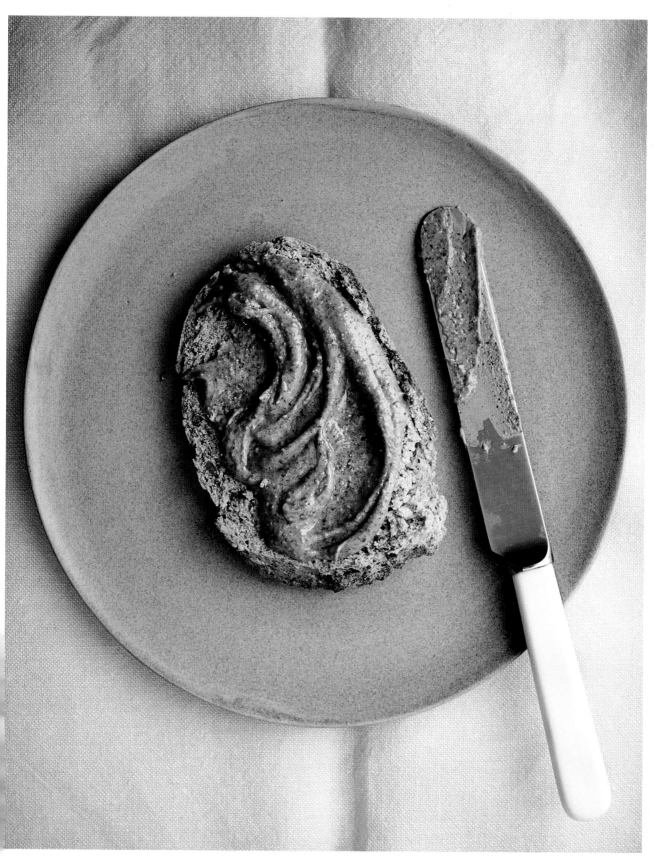

No-Knead Sourdough

Sourdough is a method of bread making that involves a fermentation process using naturally occurring *Lactobacilli* and yeast. The bread rises slowly and as a result maintains a more complex carbohydrate structure, producing a firmer loaf. The fermentation also appears to break down some of the gluten in the flour, making it easier on the gut than other bread.

Thanks to Judith Starling aka The Wild Baker for this recipe—her simple approach helps to demystify what seems like a complicated process. It is important to remember that the taste relies on many things—temperature, flour, weather, fermentation, time—and the end result is a delicious loaf of bread which reflects the environment it is raised in. This recipe uses kamut flour, an ancient grain that is high in protein and gives great depth of flavor. But you can use any whole wheat flour.

Here we assume you have a sourdough starter. You'll find more information on cleverguts.com, including how to source it online. You can make your own starter in a traditional way by using the "wild" yeast and *Lactobacilli* present in flour. Mix a small amount with water to produce the "mother," and then "feed" it with a tbsp each of flour and water over the next 3-5 days. Some people add a spoonful of active buttermilk or yogurt to help get the process underway.

Makes 1 large loaf
(about 10 slices)

2 tbsp starter

445g bread flour or
   gluten-free option

95g whole wheat bread
   flour or gluten-free option

150g kamut flour, whole
   wheat, or gluten-free flour

Salt

1 tbsp olive oil

Bread flour, for dusting

2 tbsp semolina or gluten-
   free flour, for dusting

•DAIRY-FREE OPTION

•GLUTEN-FREE OPTION

•GOOD FOR PHASE 1

The morning of the day before you want to bake your loaf, remove your starter from the fridge and refresh by feeding it with 25g bread flour, 25g whole wheat bread flour, and 50g water. Cover it with plastic wrap and leave it to proof all day at room temperature.

In the evening you should see bubbles forming on the surface or that the starter has risen, or both. Place the starter in a bowl and stir in 70g bread flour, 70g whole wheat bread flour, and 110g water—it should have a fairly thick consistency. Cover it with plastic wrap and leave it overnight. It should be clearly fermenting—thick, sticky, and bubbly. This is your "pre-ferment."

The next day, take 250g of the pre-ferment out of the bowl and place the remainder in a jar in the fridge—this will become the starter for your next loaf. Add

275ml tepid water, 150g kamut flour, 350g bread flour, and the salt to the pre-ferment in the bowl. Mix the ingredients with your hands (or in a food processor with a dough hook or a bread maker), until you have a smooth soft dough. Oil a bowl and place the dough in it and cover it with lightly oiled plastic wrap. Leave it for at least 5-6 hours at room temperature—the dough will only rise a small amount—50 percent is fine.

Once it has risen, remove it from the bowl and on a very lightly floured work surface, bring the edges of the dough to the center in a circular pattern, making a rounded loaf, and causing tension on the underside. Place the dough, seam side up, in a proofing basket dusted with a small amount of flour to prevent sticking, or use a bowl lined with a tea towel, dusted with flour. Cover it again with oiled plastic wrap and leave it to rise at room temperature for 1-3 hours.

Preheat the oven to the hottest temperature and place a baking sheet inside to heat up. Just before you are ready to bake the loaf, place a roasting pan of boiling water in the bottom of the oven (this helps to create steam). Sprinkle the semolina over the hot baking sheet (or use a sheet of reusable nonstick baking paper or silicone). Turn the loaf out onto the baking sheet and quickly slash the top with a sharp knife before putting it in the oven. Bake at 485°F for 10 minutes, then reduce the temperature to 375°F and bake for 35-40 minutes. The loaf is done if it sounds hollow when tapped underneath. Rest it on a wire rack to cool before slicing it.

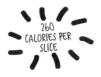

260 CALORIES PER SLICE

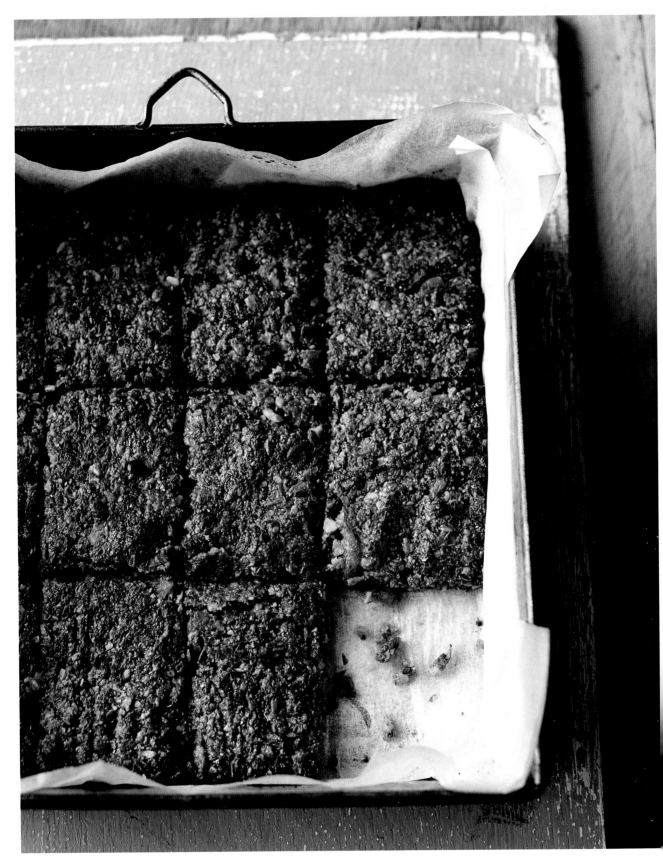

Healthy Bars and Cakes

We would encourage you to avoid snacks between meals as this brief period of "fasting" gives your body time to repair itself. As soon as you snack, any fat-burning stops and your good gut bacteria, such as *Akkermansia*, abandon their vital job of repairing the protective mucous lining of the gut wall. If you do yearn for a snack, it is best enjoyed after lunch, not only because it is digested more slowly after a meal, reducing the sugar spike, but also because you are likely to be moving around then and therefore burning the calories.

Apricot and Pistachio Bars

A tangy bar with crunchy nuts which your microbiome will love. These will keep your energy levels balanced for hours.

Makes 12
80g (½ cup) diced dates
Grated zest and juice
  of 1 orange
80g (6 tbsp) diced dried
  apricots
75g (5½ tbsp) coconut oil
160g (1⅓ cups) pistachios
Seeds from 2 cardamom
  pods
2 tbsp ground flaxseeds
¼ tsp salt

• DAIRY-FREE
• GLUTEN-FREE

1. Preheat the oven to 350°F. Line an 8-inch square baking pan with parchment paper.

2. Soften the dates by gently heating them in the orange juice and zest in a small saucepan for 2 minutes. Remove the pan from the heat and add the apricots and oil.

3. Blitz the pistachios and cardamom seeds in a food processor or with a hand blender until you have a coarse crumb. Add the date mixture, flaxseeds, and salt and pulse again.

4. Spoon the mixture into the pan and spread evenly. Bake for 20-25 minutes, until it is just starting to brown on top. Remove from the oven and allow to cool slightly in the pan before cutting into 12 bars. Store in an airtight container for up to 5 days.

190 CALORIES

Chocolate Eggplant Cake with Pear and Walnuts

Serves 8

1 medium eggplant, diced
150g (5⅓ oz) dark chocolate
  (70% cocoa), chopped
60g (4½ tbsp) coconut oil
60g (6 tbsp) chopped dates
½ tsp salt
3 eggs, beaten
1 tsp baking powder
80g (⅔ cup) ground almonds
80g (⅔ cup) chopped
  walnuts
1½ pears, cubed

•DAIRY-FREE
•GLUTEN-FREE OPTION

1. Preheat the oven to 350°F. Grease and line an 8-inch square baking pan with parchment paper.

2. Steam the eggplant for 15 minutes or until it is soft. Then place it, still hot, in a bowl. Immediately add the chocolate and oil and stir until they have more or less melted. Then mix in the dates. Blitz with a hand blender to obtain a smooth paste. Add the salt, eggs, baking powder, and almonds and whizz again, then stir in the walnuts and pears.

3. Spoon the mixture into the pan and bake for 35-40 minutes, until a knife inserted into the center comes out clean. Let cool in the pan for 10 minutes, then transfer to a wire rack.

370 CALORIES

Chocolate and Walnut Bites

Makes 16

200g (2 cups) walnuts
100g (¾ cup) pecans
75g (½ cup) raisins
225g (8 oz) pitted dates
55g (⅔ cup) cacao powder
65g (5 tbsp) coconut oil,
  melted
90g (1 cup) rolled oats
  (or gluten-free)
20g (¼ cup) desiccated
  or shredded coconut
½ tsp ground cinnamon
2 tbsp cacao nibs

•DAIRY-FREE
•GLUTEN-FREE OPTION

1. Grease and line an 8-inch square baking pan with parchment paper. Place the nuts and raisins in a bowl and cover with boiling water. Soak for 15 minutes, then drain and blitz in a food processor. Add the dates and blend again, add the cacao powder, oil, oats, coconut, and cinnamon and process until well combined.

2. Press the mixture into the pan and spread evenly. Lightly press the cacao nibs into the surface. Chill for at least 2 hours. Cut into 16 bars.

280 CALORIES

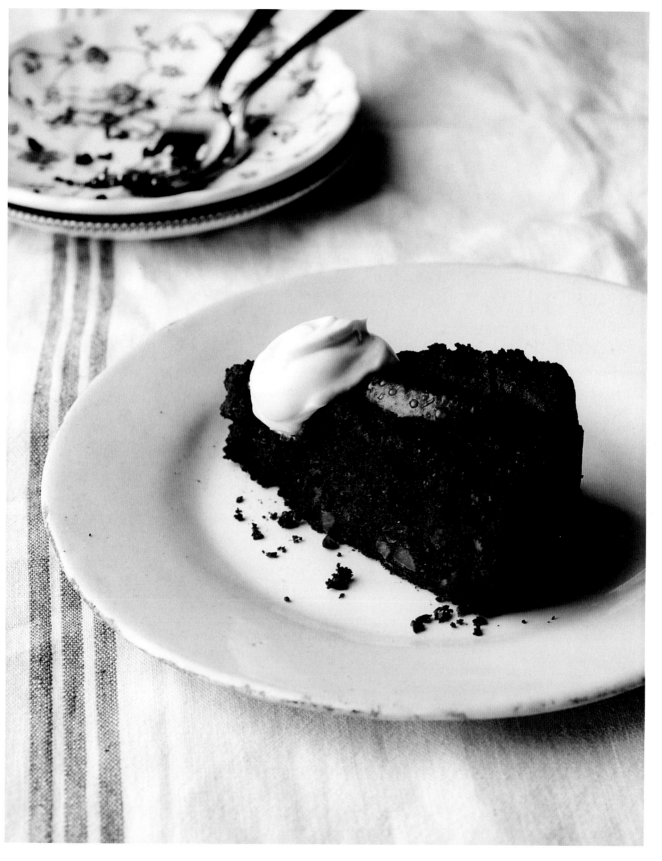

Pistachio and Olive Oil Cake

A mouthwatering cake celebrating the harmonious combination of pistachios and olive oil.

Serves 12

100g (¾ cup) dried apricot
   halves, chopped
Grated zest and juice of
   ½ lemon
2 eggs
3 tbsp extra-virgin olive oil
60g (4½ tbsp) coconut oil,
   melted
120g (1 cup) shelled
   pistachios
70g (¾ cup) ground
   almonds
1 tsp baking powder
Pinch of salt
1 tbsp honey or maple
   syrup

•DAIRY-FREE
•GLUTEN-FREE

1. Preheat the oven to 325°F. Lightly grease a 7-inch square baking pan. Place the apricots in a small saucepan along with the lemon zest and juice and 1 tbsp water. Cover the pan and simmer for a few minutes to soften the apricots, then remove them from the heat and allow them to cool.

2. Whisk the eggs in a bowl, then stir in the olive oil, coconut oil, and apricots.

3. Blitz all but about 3 tbsp of the pistachios in a food processor, add the almonds, baking powder, and salt, and pulse again. Finally, pour in the egg mixture and honey and blend.

4. Pour the mixture into the pan. Crush the remaining pistachios and sprinkle them on top. Bake the cake for 25-28 minutes, until it's golden on top and a knife inserted in the center comes out fairly clean. Leave it to rest in the pan for 10 minutes, then turn it out to cool on a wire rack.

200 CALORIES

Exotic Carrot Cake

Another deliciously moist vegetable- and nut-based cake. It doesn't melt instantly in your mouth and spike your blood sugar, but gives you a bit more to chew on, leaving enough fiber to reach your microbiome. The cardamom adds a wonderful, exotic aroma.

Serves 12

320g (11 oz) carrots, grated

80g (½ cup) finely chopped dates, or 1 tbsp honey

3 large eggs

150g (⅔ cup) coconut oil

Zest of 1 orange

Seeds from 8 cardamom pods

160g (1⅓ cups) whole wheat or buckwheat flour (or gluten-free flour)

120g (1⅓ cups) desiccated or shredded coconut, reserving 1 tbsp for scattering on top

1 tbsp baking powder

½ tsp salt

120g (1 cup) chopped walnuts

•DAIRY-FREE

•GLUTEN-FREE OPTION

1. Preheat the oven to 350°F. Grease and line an 8-inch square baking pan with parchment paper.

2. Mix the carrots, dates, eggs, coconut oil, and orange zest in a large bowl, then stir in the rest of the ingredients, except the walnuts. Blitz the mixture briefly with a hand blender or in a food processor, then vigorously stir in the nuts.

3. Pour the mixture into the pan and bake in the center of the oven for 60-75 minutes. It is done when a knife inserted in the center comes out clean. If the top is browning before the center is done, cover it with a piece of foil.

4. Scatter 1 tbsp coconut on the surface of the cake 5 minutes before removing it from the oven.

Tip: Once the pack of desiccated coconut is opened, keep it sealed in the freezer so it stays sweet and fresh.

350 CALORIES

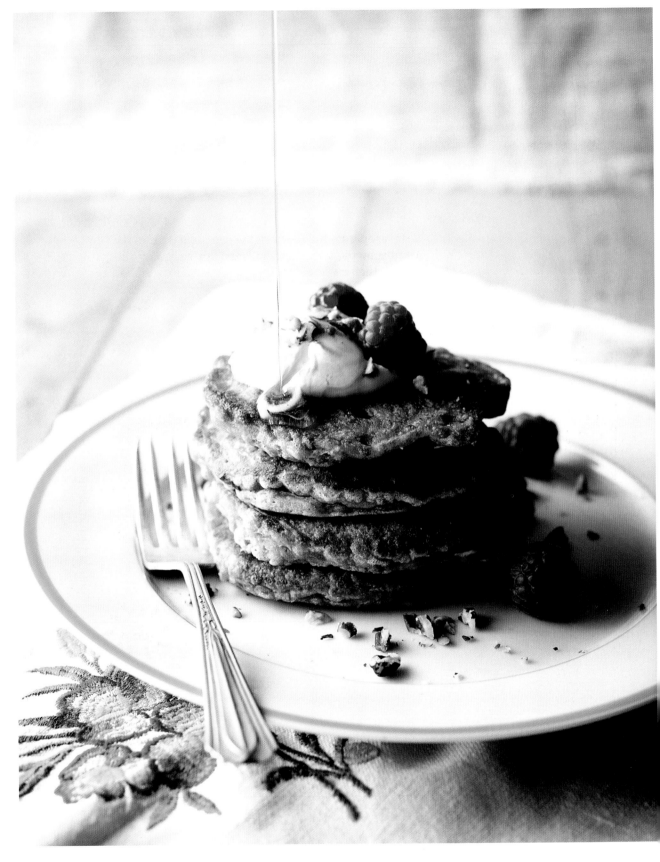

Oaty Pecan Pancakes

These indulgent whole grain pancakes have substance and flavor thanks to oats and pecans. Delicious eaten straight from the pan or, once cooled, popped in the toaster.

Makes 10-12

1½ cups gluten-free rolled oats

1 cup buckwheat flour

1 tsp ground cinnamon

1 tsp baking powder

1 pinch salt

1 egg

2 tsp vanilla extract

1 tbsp maple syrup

1 cup plus 2 tbsp almond milk (or any milk of your choice)

Scant ½ cup pecans, chopped

1 tbsp coconut oil

•DAIRY-FREE
•GLUTEN-FREE

1. Mix the oats, flour, cinnamon, baking powder, and salt in a bowl.

2. In a separate bowl, whisk the egg, then pour in the vanilla, maple syrup, and milk and stir well. Make a well in the center of the dry ingredients, pour in the wet ingredients, and gradually stir them in, followed by the nuts. The mixture should be thick but pourable. Allow it to rest for about 15 minutes.

3. Melt half the oil in a frying pan over medium heat. Drop blobs of the batter into the pan, using 1-2 tablespoonfuls for each pancake. Repeat, leaving space around each one, and cook them for 2-3 minutes, until they're golden brown and holes appear on the surface.

4. Flip them over carefully with a spatula and cook them for 1-2 minutes on the other side. Repeat with the remaining batter and oil.

5. They taste great served with 1 tbsp Greek-style yogurt (add 75 calories), 1 tsp honey (add 20 calories), and some berries or half a sliced banana (add 50 calories).

130 CALORIES

Dessert

Even a healthy microbiome can enjoy an occasional good dessert . . . though it's best to eat after a meal rather than as a snack, and avoid in Phase 1.

Kefir and Berry Fool

This fool is a great way to jazz up kefir milk, and takes minutes to assemble.

Serves 2
¾ cup kefir (see page 190)
1½ tsp xanthan gum
1 tsp vanilla extract
5 tbsp Strawberry Chia Jam
   (below)
¾ cup raspberries
⅓ cup blueberries

•GLUTEN-FREE

1. Whisk the kefir, xanthan gum, and vanilla in a bowl.

2. Layer the mixture with the jam and berries in 2 glasses.

Tip: Drizzle a little maple syrup on top if you have a sweet tooth.

Strawberry Chia Jam

Makes about 10 tbsp
2 tbsp diced dates
1 tbsp balsamic vinegar
1⅔ cups ripe strawberries,
   hulled and chopped
1 tbsp chia seeds

You will also need:
8-oz jam jar with lid

•DAIRY-FREE
•GLUTEN-FREE

1. In a medium pan, gently heat the dates with 2 tbsp water and the vinegar, stirring and pressing them with a spoon, to form a slightly lumpy paste.

2. Add the strawberries and continue to cook over low heat for 4-5 minutes, then remove the pan from the heat, add the chia seeds, and mash them into the strawberries with a spoon or masher.

3. Spoon the mixture into the jar, and once it's cool put on the lid. The jam can be stored in the fridge for up to a week.

This low-sugar chia jam is also
delicious served on the Mug Bread (page 194) or
dolloped onto oatmeal. Much loved by the microbiome,
chia seeds are made up of an astonishing 40% fiber by
weight and are a wonderful source of nutrients.

Purple Sweet Potato and Blackberry Pie

Purple sweet potatoes and blackberries are both top-of-the-range sources of soluble and insoluble fiber, and together they make a perfect pudding. The oil added here reduces the GI while increasing the absorption of nutrients, such as antioxidant carotenes. Blackberries bring a burst of fruity flavor along with a shot of vitamin C. If you can't find purple sweet potatoes, orange work well, too.

Serves 8

For the crust:

80g (⅓ cup) butter or coconut oil

20g (1½ tbsp) light muscovado sugar

120g (1¼ cups) ground almonds

100g (scant 1 cup) ground flaxseeds

30g (⅓ cup) desiccated or shredded coconut

¼ tsp Maldon sea salt

For the filling:

250g (9 oz) purple (or orange) sweet potatoes, peeled and diced

150g (5 oz) blackberries

30g (¼ cup) ground flaxseeds

60g (4½ tbsp) coconut oil

40g (¼ cup) diced dates

1 tsp vanilla extract

1 tsp ground cinnamon

1 egg

100g (3½ oz) blackberries or raspberries, for serving

•DAIRY-FREE
•GLUTEN-FREE
•GOOD FOR PHASE 1

1. Preheat the oven to 325°F. Lightly grease an 8-inch flan pan with a removable bottom.

2. For the crust: Melt the butter in a medium pan. Add the sugar and stir until it has dissolved. Remove the pan from the heat and stir in the remaining crust ingredients. Press the mixture into the bottom and sides of the pan. Bake in the middle of the oven for 20-25 minutes. The crust needs to be slightly golden and dry to the touch.

3. For the filling: Steam the sweet potatoes for 15-20 minutes, until they're soft. Then blend them thoroughly with the other filling ingredients (except the 3½ oz berries) in a food processor. Pour the mixture into the pie crust and spread it evenly.

4. Bake the pie in the middle of the oven for 15-20 minutes, until it is set in the middle and starting to turn golden brown. Allow it to cool, then scatter the blackberries on top before serving. Tastes great with a dollop of the Kefir Ginger Ice Cream (page 213).

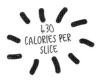

430 CALORIES PER SLICE

Dark Chocolate Avocado Mousse with Cashew Cream

A dark chocolate mousse to be eaten with a teaspoon and savored—perfect at the end of a meal. Thanks to Dara Sutin for her recipe for the delicious low-carb Cardamom Cashew Cream to drizzle over the top.

Serves 6

⅔ cup coconut cream
½ cup cocoa powder
8 soft dates, chopped
  (or 2-3 tbsp honey)
2 ripe avocados
1 tbsp coconut oil
1 tsp vanilla extract
1½ tbsp balsamic vinegar
5 oz raspberries
Cardamom Cashew Cream
  (below)

•DAIRY-FREE
•GLUTEN-FREE
•GOOD FOR PHASE 1

1. In a small saucepan, heat the coconut cream with the cocoa powder and the dates. Bring to a simmer and stir for 1-2 minutes, then set aside to cool for 5 minutes or so.

2. Pour the mixture, along with all the other ingredients, except the raspberries, into a food processor and blitz to form a smooth paste.

3. Divide the mixture among 6 teacups or glasses. Scatter the raspberries over the top. Cool the mousse in the fridge before serving with the cashew cream.

270 CALORIES

Cardamom Cashew Cream

A luxurious, versatile alternative to dairy cream.

Makes 6 portions

7 oz cashews, soaked in
  water for 2 hours
1 tsp vanilla extract
Tiny pinch of salt
1 tbsp maple syrup
Seeds from 2 cardamom
  pods

1. Drain the cashews, place them in a food processor with the vanilla, salt, maple syrup, and cardamom seeds and pulse a couple of times. Gradually add ½-⅔ cup water, blending until you have a smooth, creamy consistency.

2. Store any leftover Cashew Cream in an airtight container in the fridge for up to 3 days.

210 CALORIES

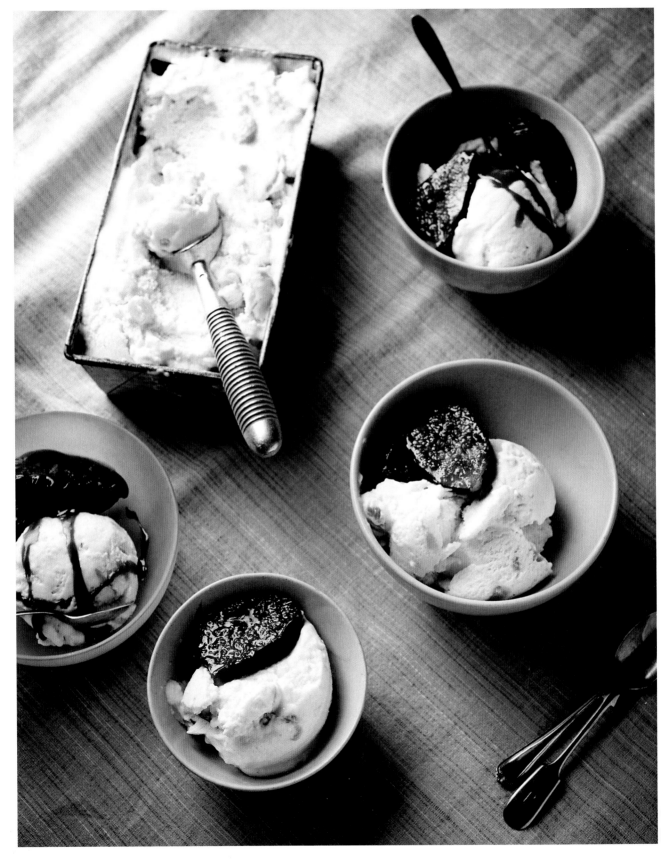

Kefir Ginger Ice Cream

This ice cream is made with active kefir cultures, which contain a far richer variety of healthy bacteria than active yogurt. Delicious served with baked or stewed fruits, such as figs, apple, or rhubarb.

Serves 4

1½ cups kefir (see page 190)

⅔ cup coconut cream

2 tsp xanthan gum

0.7 oz fresh ginger, finely diced

3 tbsp maple syrup

•GLUTEN-FREE

1. Place the kefir, coconut cream, and xanthan gum in a bowl and whisk until smooth. Vigorously mix the ginger and maple syrup in a mortar and pestle (or using a fork and a small bowl). Stir the ginger mix into the kefir, then pour the mixture into a freezer-proof container.

2. Place it in the freezer, removing it every half-hour for 2-3 hours and whisking it to break up the ice crystals. Remove it from the freezer 20-30 minutes before serving to allow it to soften.

Tip: Alternatively, use an ice-cream maker!

200 CALORIES

Red Rice Pudding

An ideal way to use up leftover rice that has already been converted to resistant starch by being cooled for 12 hours. Creamy, nutty, and exotic.

Serves 4

2 cups precooked red and brown rice

1 (14-oz) can coconut milk

¾ tsp ground cinnamon

½ tsp ground nutmeg

Seeds from 8-10 cardamom pods

1 tsp vanilla extract

1½ tbsp maple syrup

Pinch of salt

•DAIRY-FREE

•GLUTEN-FREE

•GOOD FOR PHASE 1

1. Place all the ingredients in a medium saucepan and bring to a simmer.

2. Continue to simmer, stirring occasionally, for 15 minutes, until the consistency is loose and creamy.

Note: To cook the rice in advance, cook 6 tbsp red rice and 6 tbsp brown rice in a pan of simmering water for 15-18 minutes, or until tender. Drain, refresh with cold water, then drain again. Store in the fridge for 12 hours.

330 CALORIES

Phase 1

The **Phase 1** menu plans are a guide to help ensure you have a varied diet with a good balance of nutrients during these few weeks when you are restricting ingredients. Adjust the plan to your tastes. Skip foods that you know don't suit you. This phase is mainly gluten-free and dairy-free; it is also low in beans (though vegetarians should reintroduce these after 2 weeks to maintain their protein intake).

Before you start Phase 1, we recommend you record your baseline symptoms and eating habits for at least 3 days on the Daily Food and Symptoms Diary (download from cleverguts.com).

We have generally included more substantial meals in the dinner category on the basis that many people have more time available in the evening; however, the earlier in the day that you eat your main meal, the better for weight loss, and your metabolism and microbiome. We also propose a few days when you might have a generous breakfast and skip lunch, to give your gut a brief recovery and repair period. In general, try to fast for at least 12 hours overnight.

We have not offered a menu plan for **Phase 2** (for more information on this, go to page 27), since all the recipes in this book are suitable for this phase. In Phase 2, we particularly encourage you to include more prebiotic vegetables, such as Jerusalem artichokes and chicory; and more probiotic, fermented foods such as kefir milk and Red Cabbage Sauerkraut (see chapter 6). Try to increase your consumption of multicolored vegetables and fruit and include some grains. In this phase, you get to enjoy occasional treats, too (see chapter 7).

	Breakfast	Lunch	Dinner
Monday	Simple Creamy Scrambled Eggs with smoked salmon (pg 37)	Citrus, Fennel, and Asparagus Salad (pg 55) with Turmeric Buttermilk Dressing (pg 119)	Baked Coconut Chicken Curry (pg 126) with 2 tbsp Red Rice with Resistant Starch (pg 176) and steamed leafy greens
Tuesday	Blueberry Chia Pot (pg 45) with 1 tbsp berries	Green Gazpacho with Seaweed (pg 63)	Prosciutto-Wrapped Pork Loin (pg 149) with Creamy Nutmeg Spinach (pg 160)
Wednesday	Turmeric Spiced Omelet with Seaweed (pg 38)	Smoked Salmon Ceviche (pg 84) with Thai-Flavored Seaweed Crackers (pg 79)	Bitter Greens and Toasted Pine Nut Salad (pg 56) with Apple Cider Vinegar Dressing (pg 117), followed by Michael's Mussels (pg 98)
Thursday	Coconut Oatmeal with Pecans and Pear (pg 42)	Crab Spaghetti with Seaweed (pg 101)	Steak with Guacamole and Blistered Tomatoes (pg 153)
Friday	Sour Cream and Seaweed Muffin (pg 83)	Chinese Noodle Jar (pg 70)	Baked Salmon with Seaweed Pesto (pg 132) and Beets Roasted in Their Skins (pg 170)
Saturday	Bircher Muesli with Kefir (pg 45)	Skip lunch	Beef and Orange Stew with Mushrooms (pg 150) with Pan-Fried Zucchini Spaghetti (pg 177)
Sunday	Simple Creamy Scrambled Eggs (pg 37) with avocado	Mackerel with Quinoa Tabbouleh (pg 106)	Easy Chicken Tagine with Preserved Lemon (pg 127) and Red Rice with Resistant Starch (pg 176)

	Breakfast	Lunch	Dinner
Monday	Simple Creamy Scrambled Eggs with smoked salmon (pg 37)	Phyto Salad (pg 66)	Vegetable and Paneer Curry (pg 145) with 1 tbsp Greek yogurt and 2 tbsp cooked, cooled, and reheated brown rice
Tuesday	Coconut Oatmeal with Pecans and Pears (pg 42)	Turkey and Mushroom Bolognese (pg 131) with Pan-Fried Zucchini Spaghetti (pg 177)	Turmeric Coronation Chicken (pg 111), Cauliflower Rice with Cilantro (pg 174), and steamed leafy greens
Wednesday	Avocado and Smoked Salmon (pg 46)	Terra Mare Salad (pg 88) with 2 tbsp quinoa	Marinated Tofu Stir-Fry with Noodles (pg 144)
Thursday	Yogurt with Chia Jam and Toasted Pistachios (pg 35)	Pasta with Pistachio Pesto (pg 99) with Citrus, Fennel, and Asparagus Salad (page 55) or steamed vegetables	Thai Shrimp with Coconut Milk and Seaweed (pg 141) with 2 tbsp cooked, cooled, and reheated brown rice
Friday	Creamy Pineapple Smoothie (pg 51)	Tuna and Vegetable Stir-Fry with Seaweed (pg 109)	Michael's Mussels (pg 98) with 2 slices of Mug Bread (pg 194)
Saturday	Full English Breakfast with Green Bananas (pg 41)	Healing Chicken Bone Broth (pg 59)	Lazy Lemon and Lime Chicken (pg 130) and Creamy Nutmeg Spinach (pg 160)
Sunday	Simple Creamy Scrambled Eggs (pg 37) with fried mushrooms	Skip lunch	Seafood with Seaweed Risotto (pg 139) with Quick Garlic-Fried Greens (pg 161)

	Breakfast	Lunch	Dinner
Monday	Dr. Tim's Healthy Gut Smoothie (pg 50)	Citrus, Fennel, and Asparagus Salad (pg 55) with Avocado and Lime Salsa (pg 75)	Veira's Cilantro Chicken (pg 128) with Spinach Dal (pg 112) and 2 tbsp quinoa
Tuesday	Simple Creamy Scrambled Eggs with leafy greens and Parmesan (pg 37)	Smoked Salmon Ceviche with a leafy green salad (pg 84)	Mackerel Fillets with Spiced Coconut (pg 133) and Beets Roasted in Their Skins (pg 170) and steamed leafy greens
Wednesday	Kale and Tofu Scramble (pg 93)	Warm Red Rice Salad with Zucchini (pg 90)	Sea Bass with Seaweed Salsa Verde (pg 135) and Roasted Butternut Squash (pg 172)
Thursday	Clever Gut Green Smoothie (pg 48)	Pink Celeriac and Beet Soup (pg 64) with Flaxseed Crackers (pg 78)	Black Bean Beet Burger (pg 147) with Quick Garlic-Fried Greens (pg 161) and 2 tbsp quinoa
Friday	Turmeric Spiced Omelet with Seaweed (pg 38)	Crab Spaghetti with Seaweed (pg 101) with steamed green and colored vegetables	Bitter Greens and Toasted Pine Nut Salad (pg 56) with Apple Cider Vinegar Dressing (pg 117) followed by Mackerel with Quinoa Tabbouleh (pg 106)
Saturday	Coconut Oatmeal with Pecans and Pears (pg 42)	Poor Man's Potatoes with Anchovies (pg 102)	Easy Chicken Tagine with Preserved Lemon (pg 127) with Roasted Butternut Squash (pg 172)
Sunday	Simple Creamy Scrambled Eggs (pg 37) with Slow-Roasted Tomatoes (pg 172)	Green Banana and Pepper Stir-Fry (pg 163)	Bitter Green Salad (page 56) followed by Sweet Potato, Kale, and Cod Fishcakes (pg 136) and Eggplant Chips (pg 175)

	Breakfast	Lunch	Dinner
Monday	Blueberry Chia Pot (pg 45)	Phyto Salad (pg 66)	Turmeric Coronation Chicken (pg 111) with Red Rice with Resistant Starch (pg 176) and steamed vegetables
Tuesday	Clever Gut Green Smoothie (pg 48)	Smoked Mackerel and Kale Kedgeree (pg 47) with Slow-Roasted Tomatoes (pg 172)	Eggplant Parmigiana (pg 96) with steamed colored and dark leafy greens
Wednesday	Simple Creamy Scrambled Eggs (pg 37) with cremini mushrooms	Bitter Greens and Toasted Pine Nut Salad (pg 56) with Lime Dressing (pg 116)	Marinated Tofu Stir-Fry with Noodles (pg 144)
Thursday	Yogurt with Chia Jam and Toasted Pistachios (pg 35)	Roasted Mediterranean Vegetables, Pearl Barley, and Eggs (pg 105)	Sausage and Mediterranean Sheet Pan Bake (pg 154) with 2 tbsp brown rice or quinoa
Friday	Bircher Muesli made with nondairy milk (pg 45)	Pistachio Pesto (pg 99) with Quick Garlic-Fried Greens (pg 161)	Squid Provençal (pg 142) with 2 tbsp brown rice or quinoa
Saturday	Full English Breakfast with Green Bananas (pg 41)	Skip lunch	Turkey and Mushroom Bolognese (pg 131) with Pan-Fried Zucchini Spaghetti (pg 177)
Sunday	Creamy Pineapple Smoothie (pg 51)	Spicy Lentil and Tomato Soup (pg 62) with Flaxseed Crackers (pg 78)	Beef and Orange Stew with Mushrooms (pg 150) with Cauliflower Baked with Lemon and Almonds (pg 95) and steamed greens

Planner for 5:2 Days (800 calories a day)

Feel free to swap the lunch and dinner menus. Steamed greens or crudités add only a few extra calories and contribute fiber, so feel free to add them. If skipping a meal is difficult, have some Quick Seaweed Miso Soup (page 61) or Gut-Soothing Vegetable Bouillon (page 60) to tide you over.

Breakfast	Lunch	Dinner	Calories
Simple Creamy Scrambled Eggs with smoked salmon (280 cal, pg 37)	Skip lunch	Easy Chicken Tagine with Preserved Lemon (470 cal, pg 127) and Red Rice with Resistant Starch (90 cal, pg 176)	840
Turmeric Spiced Omelet with Seaweed (270 cal, pg 38)	Pink Celeriac and Beet Soup (210 cal, pg 64)	Mackerel with Quinoa Tabbouleh (410 cal, pg 106)	890
Yogurt with Chia Jam and Toasted Pistachios (230 cal, pg 35)	Grilled Red Pepper Dip (160 cal, pg 73) with cucumber crudités	Steak with Guacamole and Blistered Tomatoes (470 cal, pg 153)	860
Avocado and Smoked Salmon (280 cal, pg 46)	Skip lunch	Lazy Lemon and Lime Chicken (560 cal, pg 130) with steamed greens	840
Simple Creamy Scrambled Eggs with smoked salmon (280 cal, pg 37)	Tuna and Vegetable Stir-Fry with Seaweed (580 cal, pg 109)	Roasted Butternut Squash (240 cal, pg 172) and Scorched Purple Radicchio (10 cal, pg 160)	800
Creamy Pineapple Smoothie (460 cal, pg 51)	Quick Seaweed Miso Soup (15 cal, pg 61) with 1 Thai-Flavored Seaweed Cracker (160 cal, pg 79)	Bitter Greens and Toasted Pine Nut Salad (260 cal, pg 56)	800
Simple Creamy Scrambled Eggs (190 cal, pg 37)	Quick Garlic-Fried Greens (290 cal, pg 161)	Quorn and Parsnip Shepherd's Pie (410 cal, pg 148)	890
Sour Cream and Seaweed Muffin (200 cal, pg 83)	2 Spinach and Ricotta Blinis (240 cal, pg 80) with half serving of Smoked Mackerel Pâté (80 cal, pg 75)	Brazilian-Style Crab (370 cal, pg 110) with steamed greens	890
Simple Creamy Scrambled Eggs (190 cal, pg 37)	Citrus, Fennel, and Asparagus Salad (100 cal, pg 55) with Turmeric Buttermilk Dressing (70 cal, pg 119)	Prosciutto-Wrapped Pork Loin (420 cal, pg 149) Red Rice with Resistant Starch (90 cal, pg 176)	870
Dr. Tim's Healthy Gut Smoothie (520 cal, pg 50)	Skip lunch	Sea Bass with Seaweed Salsa Verde (380 cal, pg 135) and steamed greens	900
1 Spinach and Ricotta Blini (120 cal, pg 80) with slice smoked salmon (90 cal)	Quick Seaweed Miso Soup (15 cal, pg 61), Flaxseed Cracker (80 cal, pg 78)	Sausage and Mediterranean Sheet Pan Bake (510 cal, pg 154)	820
Simple Creamy Scrambled Eggs (190 cal, pg 37)	Spicy Lentil and Tomato Soup (160 cal, pg 62)	Sweet Potato, Kale, and Cod Fishcakes (340 cal, pg 136) and Citrus, Fennel, and Asparagus Salad (100 cal, pg 55) with Lemony Buttermilk Dressing (70 cal, pg 118)	860
1 Apricot and Pistachio Bar (190 cal, pg 201)	Smoked Mackerel Pàté (160 cal, pg 75) with 2 Flaxseed Crackers (160 cal, pg 78)	Green Beans and Edamame with Anchovies (240 cal, pg 87)	780
Clever Gut Green Smoothie (450 cal, pg 48)	Skip lunch	Smoked Salmon Ceviche (450 cal, pg 84)	900
1 Oaty Pecan Pancake (130 cal, pg 207)	Chinese Noodle Jar (300 cal, pg 70)	Tofu Stir-Fry with Noodles (410 cal, pg 144)	840

Acknowledgments

I am hugely appreciative to Michael for involving me in the exciting new world of gut health and for testing some strange concoctions with good humor and wise advice. Likewise, thanks to all four children, Alex, Jack, Dan, and Kate, for their encouragement and honest feedback(!). And particularly for the invaluable insights from one who turned out to be gluten-intolerant during the writing of the book and remains happily gluten-free.

Special thanks to Rebecca Nicolson and the rest of the talented team at Short Books; editor Aurea Carpenter for her vision, turn of phrase, and excellent guidance; Paul Bougourd; and Andrew Smith for his design.

A big thank you to consultant nutritionist Joy Skipper for testing, advising, contributing delicious recipes, and ensuring all is nutritionally sound, and also to Sue Camp for excellent advice and recipe analysis.

The wonderful, luscious images were created by photographer Joe Sarah and food stylist Dara Sutin.

Thanks also to friends and family who have patiently answered endless questions about traditional cooking, recipes, and fermentation, including my niece Emily, an expert in Japanese food; mother-in-law Joan; stepmother Wendy; brother Aidan; sisters-in-law Nikki and Sylvia; and great friend, cook, and ferment soulmate, Caroline Barton. Also to my mother, a superb and adventurous cook, who celebrated food, taught us to cook, and would have loved to have been involved.

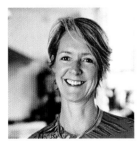

Dr. Clare Bailey is a general practitioner doing diet research with Oxford University. She is the author of *The 8-Week Blood Sugar Diet Cookbook*, and is married to Dr. Michael Mosley, author of *The Clever Gut Diet*, *The FastDiet*, and *The 8-Week Blood Sugar Diet*. She is also founder of Parenting Matters, an organization that helps parents become more confident through courses and one-on-one consultations.

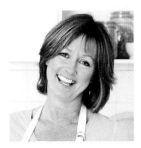

Joy Skipper is a qualified nutritionist who has worked in the food industry for over twenty years, writing cookbooks and advising clients on healthy diet and lifestyle.

Index

5:2 diet 11, 19, 217

abdominal fat 22
activity 22
Akkermansia 18, 201
allergic diseases 6, 23
almonds
 cauliflower baked with lemon
  and almonds 95
 eggplant chips 175
 mug bread 194
amino acids 106
anchovies
 anchovy and rosemary dressing
  116
 green beans and edamame with
  anchovies 87
 poor man's potatoes and
  anchovies 102
 salsa verde with seaweed 117
 shrimp with pasta and seaweed
  138
antibiotics 6
antioxidants 14, 94
appetite 20
apple cider vinegar
 beef and orange stew with
  mushrooms 150
 bitter greens and toasted pine
  nut salad 56
 chicken bone broth 59
 cider vinegar aperitif 56
 dressing 117
 green gazpacho with seaweed
  63
 Japanese-style quick-pickled
  vegetables 167
 nutrition 17, 56
 Quorn and parsnip shepherd's
  pie 148
 salsa verde with seaweed 117
apricots
 apricot and pistachio bars 201
 easy chicken tagine with
  preserved lemons 127
 healthy homemade granola 34
 pistachio and olive oil cake 204
 turmeric coronation chicken 111
asparagus
 broccoli and asparagus with
  buttermilk dressing 90
 citrus, fennel, and asparagus
  salad 55
avocado
 avocado and lime salsa 75
 avocado and smoked salmon 46
 clever gut green smoothie 48
 dark chocolate avocado mousse
  with cashew cream 211
 Dr. Tim's healthy gut smoothie 50

phyto salad lunchbox 69
smoked salmon ceviche 84
steak with guacamole and
 blistered tomatoes 153

bacon, full English breakfast
 with green bananas 41
bananas
 full English breakfast with
  green bananas 41
 green banana and pepper
  stir-fry 163
bean sprouts, marinated tofu
 stir-fry with noodles 144
beans
 black bean beet burgers 147
 smoky eggplant and
  cannellini beans 164
beef
 beef and orange stew with
  mushrooms 150
 steak with guacamole and
  blistered tomatoes 153
beets
 beet and chile spread 77
 beet and yogurt dip 72
 beets roasted in their skins 170
 black bean beet burgers 147
 mackerel with quinoa
  tabbouleh 106
 pink celeriac and beet soup 64
berries
 kefir and berry fool 208
 yogurt with chia jam and
  toasted pistachios 35
bhajis, onion and zucchini 162
bircher muesli with kefir 45
bitter greens and toasted pine nut
 salad 56
black bean beet burgers 147
blackberries, purple sweet potato
 and blackberry pie 210
blinis, spinach and ricotta 80
blood orange salad with toasted
 coriander 55
blood sugar 18, 19, 20, 59
blue cheese butter 121
blueberries
 blueberry chia pots 45
 clever gut green smoothie 48
 Dr. Tim's healthy gut smoothie 50
bok choy, Dr. Tim's healthy gut
 smoothie 50
bouillon, vegetable 60
Brazilian-style crab 110
breads
 mug bread 194
 no-knead sourdough 198–9
 seeded soda bread 196
 whole grain flatbread 195

breakfast 20
 full English breakfast with
  green bananas 41
broccoli
 and asparagus with buttermilk
  dressing 90
 low-carb mac 'n' cheese 92
 marinated tofu stir-fry with
  noodles 144
 Thai shrimp with coconut milk
  and seaweed 141
 toasted slaw with halloumi and
  lemony buttermilk dressing 89
broth, healing chicken bone
 broth 59
buttermilk
 lemony buttermilk dressing 118
 nutrition 54
 sour cream and seaweed
  muffins 83
 toasted slaw with halloumi and
  lemony buttermilk dressing 89
 turmeric buttermik dressing 119
butternut squash
 pasta with pistachio pesto 99
 Quorn and parsnip shepherd's
  pie 148
 roasted 172
 roasted Mediterranean
  vegetables, pearl barley, and
  eggs 105
 turkey and mushroom
  bolognese 131
butters, flavored 121

cabbage
 full English breakfast with green
  bananas 41
 mushroom omelet with red
  sauerkraut 38
 red cabbage sauerkraut 185
 toasted slaw with halloumi and
  lemony buttermilk dressing
  89
 tuna and vegetable stir-fry with
  seaweed 109
 warm red rice salad with
  zucchini 90
cakes
 chocolate eggplant cake
  202
 exotic carrot cake 205
 pistachio and olive oil cake
  204
calorie intake 11
cannellini beans, with smoky
 eggplant 164
carbohydrates, starchy 10
cardamom cashew cream 211
carotenoids 67

carrots
  beef and orange stew with
    mushrooms 150
  exotic carrot cake 205
  gut-soothing vegetable bouillon
    60
  healing chicken bone broth 59
  mackerel with quinoa
    tabbouleh 106
  roasted purple carrots with
    tarragon 171
  turkey and mushroom
    bolognese 131
cashews
  bircher muesli with kefir 45
  cardamom cashew cream 211
  chickpea, coconut, and cashew
    curry 107
  Chinese noodle jar 70
  creamy pineapple smoothie 51
  dark chocolate avocado mousse
    with cashew cream 211
  marinated tofu stir-fry with
    noodles 144
cauliflower
  baked with lemon and almonds
    95
  broccoli and asparagus with
    buttermilk dressing 90
  cauliflower rice with cilantro
    174
  low-carb mac 'n' cheese 92
  smoked mackerel and kale
    kedgeree 47
  vegetable and paneer curry 145
celeriac
  pink celeriac and beet soup 64
  Quorn and parsnip shepherd's
    pie 148
celery
  beef and orange stew with
    mushrooms 150
  chickpea, coconut, and cashew
    curry 107
  clever gut green smoothie 48
  gut-soothing vegetable bouillon
    60
  healing chicken bone broth 59
  shrimp with pasta and seaweed
    138
  tuna and vegetable stir-fry with
    seaweed 109
  Veira's cilantro chicken with
    yogurt and fennel 128
celiac disease 23
ceviche, smoked salmon 84
cheese
  black bean beet burgers 147
  blue cheese butter 121
  broccoli and asparagus with
    buttermilk dressing 90
  eggplant parmigiana 96
  low-carb mac 'n' cheese 92
  pasta with pistachio pesto 99

roasted Mediterranean
  vegetables, pearl barley, and
  eggs 105
simple creamy scrambled eggs
  with leafy greens and
  Parmesan 37
sour cream and seaweed
  muffins 83
spinach dal 112
toasted slaw with halloumi and
  lemony buttermilk dressing
  89
vegetable and paneer curry
  145
warm lentil salad 87
chia seeds
  blueberry chia pots 45
  flaxseed crackers 78
  nutrition 209
  seeded soda bread 196
  strawberry chia jam 208
  yogurt with chia jam and
    toasted pistachios 35
chicken
  coconut chicken curry, baked
    126
  lazy lemon and lime chicken
    130
  tagine with preserved lemons
    127
  turmeric coronation chicken
    111
  Veira's cilantro chicken with
    yogurt and fennel 128
chicken bone broth 59
chickpeas
  chickpea, coconut, and cashew
    curry 107
  lemon-cilantro hummus
    with seaweed 74
Chinese noodle jar 70
chocolate and walnut bites 202
chocolate avocado mousse with
  cashew cream 211
chocolate eggplant cake 202
citrus, fennel, and asparagus
  salad 55
Clever Gut diet
  phase one 25, 214–16
  phase two 27
coconut, dry sambal 120
coconut cream
  dark chocolate avocado mousse
    with cashew cream 211
  kefir ginger ice cream 213
coconut milk
  baked coconut chicken curry
    126
  blueberry chia pots 45
  Brazilian-style crab 110
  chickpea, coconut, and cashew
    curry 107
  coconut oatmeal with pecans
    and pear 42

red rice pudding 213
spinach dal 112
Thai shrimp with coconut milk
  and seaweed 141
cod, sweet potato, kale, and cod
  fishcakes 136
coronation chicken, turmeric 111
cortisol 22
crab
  Brazilian-style crab 110
  crab spaghetti with seaweed 101
crackers
  flaxseed 78
  Thai-flavored seaweed 79
cranberries
  bircher muesli with kefir 45
  healthy homemade granola 34
cream cheese spreads 77
creamy pesto dressing 119
cruciferous vegetables 94
curcumin 17, 111
curries
  baked coconut chicken curry
    126
  chickpea, coconut, and cashew
    curry 107
  spinach dal 112
  vegetable and paneer curry 145

dal, spinach 112
dairy foods 12–13, 27, 77
dark chocolate avocado mousse
  with cashew cream 211
dates
  apricot and pistachio bars 201
  chocolate and walnut bites 202
  dark chocolate avocado mousse
    with cashew cream 211
  exotic carrot cake 205
  healthy homemade granola 34
  purple sweet potato and
    blackberry pie 210
  strawberry chia jam 208
diabetes, type 2 6, 10, 19, 66
diary keeping 24, 27
digestive enzyme production 11
dips
  beet and yogurt 72
  grilled red pepper 73
dressings
  anchovy and rosemary 116
  apple cider vinegar 117
  creamy pesto kefir 119
  kefir mustard 119
  lemony buttermilk 118
  lime 116
  salsa verde with seaweed 117
  turmeric buttermilk 119
drinks 19
  clever gut green smoothie 48
  creamy pineapple smoothie 51
  Dr. Tim's healthy gut smoothie 50
  kombucha 180–2
  turmeric tea 21

edamame beans
  Chinese noodle jar 70
  green beans and edamame with
    anchovies 87
  pea and edamame mash 162
  smoked salmon ceviche 84
eggplant 24
  chocolate eggplant cake 202
  eggplant chips 175
  eggplant parmigiana 96
  roasted Mediterranean
    vegetables, pearl barley, and
    eggs 105
  smoky eggplant and cannellini
    beans 164
  vegetable and paneer curry
    145
eggs
  mushroom omelet with red
    sauerkraut 38
  nutrition 17
  roasted Mediterranean
    vegetables, pearl barley, and
    eggs 105
  scrambled 37
  smoked mackerel and kale
    kedgeree 47
  spinach and ricotta blinis 80
  turmeric spiced omelet with
    seaweed 38
exclusion diets 13
exercise 22

fats 12, 17
fennel
  citrus, fennel, and asparagus
    salad 55
  prosciutto-wrapped pork loin
    149
  shrimp with pasta and seaweed
    138
  Veira's cilantro chicken with
    yogurt and fennel 128
fermented foods 8, 14, 17
fiber 13–14
fish
  anchovy and rosemary dressing
    116
  avocado and smoked salmon
    46
  baked salmon with seaweed
    pesto 132
  green beans and edamame with
    anchovies 87
  mackerel fillets with spiced
    coconut 133
  mackerel with quinoa
    tabbouleh 106
  nutrition 12, 17, 46
  phyto salad lunchbox 69
  poor man's potatoes with
    anchovies 102
  sea bass with seaweed salsa
    verde 135

smoked mackerel and kale
    kedgeree 47
  smoked mackerel pâté 75
  smoked salmon ceviche 84
  smoked salmon spread 77
  sweet potato, kale, and cod
    fishcakes 136
  tuna and vegetable stir-fry with
    seaweed 109
flavonoids 67
flaxseed crackers 78
flour 13
FODMAPs 24
food allergies 23
food intolerances 6, 12, 23, 25
food labels 10
fructooligosaccharides 14
fruit, variety 14, 17

garlic and parsley butter 121
gazpacho, green with seaweed
    63
gluten 13, 27
Glycemic Index (GI) 10
grains 13
granola
  healthy homemade 34
  with yogurt and pear 32
green beans and edamame with
    anchovies 87
greens, quick garlic-fried 161
gut lining 18, 201

halloumi, toasted slaw with
    halloumi and lemony buttermilk
    dressing 89
healing chicken bone broth 59
herb butter 121
horseradish spread 77
hummus, lemon-cilantro with
    seaweed 74

IBS 14, 23, 24
ice cream, kefir ginger 213
immune system 22
inflammation 10, 24
ingredient planning 28–9
insulin 12
intermittent fasting (IF) 18 see
    also 5:2 diet
inulin 14, 20

Japanese-style quick-pickled
    vegetables 167
Jerusalem artichokes, roasted
    171

kale
  clever gut green smoothie 48
  full English breakfast with
    green bananas 41
  kale and tofu scramble 93
  smoked mackerel and kale
    kedgeree 47

sweet potato, kale, and cod
    fishcakes 136
kefir
  bircher muesli with kefir 45
  creamy pesto kefir dressing
    119
  kefir and berry fool 208
  kefir ginger ice cream 213
  kefir milk 190–1
  kefir mustard dressing 119
  seeded soda bread 196
kombucha 180–2

Lactobacillus 17, 189, 198
lactose intolerance 12–13
lamb, slow-roasted shoulder 157
leaky gut syndrome 24
leeks
  gut-soothing vegetable bouillon
    60
  healing chicken bone broth 59
  terra mare salad 88
lemons
  cauliflower baked with lemon
    and almonds 95
  easy chicken tagine with
    preserved lemons 127
  lazy lemon and lime chicken
    130
  lemon and pepper butter 121
  lemon-cilantro hummus
    with seaweed 74
  lemony buttermilk dressing
    118
  preserved 184
  terra mare salad 88
  warm red rice salad with
    zucchini 90
lentils
  Puy lentils with balsamic
    vinegar 169
  spicy lentil and tomato soup 62
  spinach dal 112
  warm lentil salad 87
limes
  avocado and lime salsa 75
  Brazilian-style crab 110
  chickpea, coconut, and cashew
    curry 107
  dry coconut sambal 120
  lazy lemon and lime chicken
    130
  lime dressing 116
  smoked salmon ceviche 84
  Thai shrimp with coconut milk
    and seaweed 141
low-carb mac 'n' cheese 92

mac 'n' cheese, low-carb 92
mackerel
  mackerel fillets with spiced
    coconut 133
  mackerel with quinoa
    tabbouleh 106

mackerel (*cont.*)
  smoked mackerel and kale
    kedgeree 47
  smoked mackerel pâté 75
meal plans 214–17
meat 12, 149, 157
medical checks 23
Mediterranean style food 10
Mediterranean vegetables, pearl
  barley, and eggs, roasted 105
metabolism 22
microbiome 6, 8, 22
milk
  Dr. Tim's healthy gut smoothie 50
  kefir 190–1
mindfulness 22
miso
  Chinese noodle jar 70
  quick seaweed miso soup 61
muffins, sour cream and seaweed
  83
mug bread 194
mushrooms
  beef and orange stew with
    mushrooms 150
  cremini, with scrambled eggs 37
  full English breakfast with
    green bananas 41
  lazy lemon and lime chicken
    130
  mushroom omelet with red
    sauerkraut 38
  toasted slaw with halloumi and
    lemony buttermilk dressing 89
  turkey and mushroom
    Bolognese 131
mussels, Michael's 98
mustard butter 121
mustard seeds 94

nightshade vegetables 24
noodles
  Chinese noodle jar 70
  marinated tofu stir-fry with
    noodles 144
nuts
  apricot and pistachio bars 201
  bircher muesli with kefir 45
  blueberry chia pots 45
  cardamom cashew cream 211
  cauliflower baked with lemon
    and almonds 95
  chickpea, coconut, and cashew
    curry 107
  Chinese noodle jar 70
  chocolate and walnut bites
    202
  chocolate avocado mousse with
    cashew cream 211
  chocolate eggplant cake 202
  coconut oatmeal with pecans
    and pear 42
  eggplant chips 175
  exotic carrot cake 205

marinated tofu stir-fry with
  noodles 144
mug bread 194
nut butter 123
nutrition 17
oaty pecan pancakes 207
pasta with pistachio pesto 99
pistachio and olive oil cake 204
yogurt with chia jam and
  toasted pistachios 35

oats
  bircher muesli with kefir 45
  chocolate and walnut bites 202
  coconut oatmeal with pecans
    and pear 42
  healthy homemade granola 34
  oaty pecan pancakes 207
obesity 6
olive oil
  nutrition 17
  pistachio and olive oil cake 204
omega-3 fatty acids 46
omelet
  mushroom, with red sauerkraut
    38
  turmeric spiced, with seaweed
    38
onions
  avocado and lime salsa 75
  baked salmon with seaweed
    pesto 132
  blood orange salad with toasted
    coriander 55
  broccoli and asparagus with
    buttermilk dressing 90
  chickpea, coconut, and cashew
    curry 107
  gut-soothing vegetable bouillon
    60
  healing chicken bone broth 59
  lazy lemon and lime chicken
    130
  onion and zucchini bhajis 162
  poor man's potatoes with
    anchovies 102
  red cabbage sauerkraut 185
  sausage and Mediterranean
    vegetable sheet pan bake 154
  smoked mackerel and kale
    kedgeree 47
  spicy pickled 189
  squid Provençal 142
  tuna and vegetable stir-fry with
    seaweed 109
  vegetable and paneer curry 145
  warm lentil salad 87
oranges
  beef and orange stew with
    mushrooms 150
  blood orange salad with toasted
    coriander 55
  citrus, fennel, and asparagus
    salad 55

palate 11
pancetta, full English breakfast
  with green bananas 41
pantry ingredients 28–9
parsnips, Quorn and parsnip
  shepherd's pie 148
pasta
  crab spaghetti with seaweed
    101
  low-carb mac 'n' cheese 92
  pasta with pistachio pesto 99
  shrimp with pasta and seaweed
    138
  Thai shrimp with coconut milk
    and seaweed 141
pâté, smoked mackerel 75
pea and edamame mash 162
pearl barley, roasted
  Mediterranean vegetables, pearl
    barley, and eggs 105
pears
  chocolate eggplant cake
    202
  coconut oatmeal with pecans
    and pear 42
  yogurt with granola and diced
    pear 32
pecans
  blueberry chia pots 45
  chocolate and walnut bites 202
  coconut oatmeal with pecans
    and pear 42
  oaty pecan pancakes 207
peppers (bell) 24
  baked coconut chicken curry
    126
  baked salmon with seaweed
    pesto 132
  Brazilian-style crab 110
  easy chicken tagine with
    preserved lemon 127
  green banana and pepper stir-
    fry 163
  grilled red pepper dip 73
  marinated tofu stir-fry with
    noodles 144
  poor man's potatoes with
    anchovies 102
  roasted Mediterranean
    vegetables, pearl barley, and
    eggs 105
  sausage and Mediterranean
    vegetable sheet pan bake 154
  smoked mackerel and kale
    kedgeree 47
  squid Provençal 142
  tuna and vegetable stir-fry with
    seaweed 109
  vegetable and paneer curry 145
pesto
  baked salmon with seaweed
    pesto 132
  creamy pesto kefir dressing 119
  pasta with pistachio pesto 99

phyto salad 66–7
phyto salad lunchbox 69
phytonutrients 14, 67
pie, purple sweet potato and
    blackberry 210
pine nuts
    bitter greens and toasted pine
        nut salad 56
    mackerel with quinoa
        tabbouleh 106
    warm red rice salad with
        zucchini 90
pineapple, creamy pineapple
    smoothie 51
pistachios
    apricot and pistachio bars 201
    pasta with pistachio pesto 99
    pistachio and olive oil cake
        204
    yogurt with chia jam and
        toasted pistachios 35
planning 19, 20, 214–17
polyphenols 14, 67
pork, prosciutto-wrapped pork
    loin 149
portion control 20
potatoes 24
    baked 11
    poor man's potatoes with
        anchovies 102
prebiotics 14, 27, 40
probiotics 8, 14, 27, 54
processed foods 10
prosciutto-wrapped pork loin
    149
protein
    intake 12, 157
    variety 8, 12
Puy lentils with balsamic vinegar
    169

quick seaweed miso soup 61
quinoa
    black bean beet burgers 147
    lazy lemon and lime chicken
        130
    mackerel with quinoa
        tabbouleh 106
    phyto salad lunchbox 69
    terra mare salad 88
Quorn and parsnip shepherd's
    pie 148

radicchio, scorched purple
    160
red peppers, see peppers (bell)
resistant starch 40, 41, 176
riboflavin 106
rice
    red rice pudding 213
    red rice with resistant starch
        176
    seafood with seaweed risotto
        139

smoked mackerel and kale
    kedgeree 47
warm red rice salad with
    zucchini 90
ricotta, spinach and ricotta blinis
    80

salads
    bitter greens and toasted pine
        nut salad 56
    blood orange salad with toasted
        coriander 55
    citrus, fennel, and asparagus
        salad 55
    phyto salad 66–7
    phyto salad lunchbox 69
    smoked salmon ceviche 84
    terra mare salad 88
    toasted slaw with halloumi and
        lemony buttermilk dressing
        89
    warm lentil salad 87
    warm red rice salad with
        zucchini 90
salmon
    avocado and smoked salmon
        46
    baked salmon with seaweed
        pesto 132
    phyto salad lunchbox 69
    smoked salmon ceviche 84
    smoked salmon spread 77
salsas
    avocado and lime salsa 75
    salsa verde with seaweed 117
sambal, dry coconut 120
satiety 19
sauerkraut
    mushroom omelet with red
        sauerkraut 38
    red cabbage sauerkraut 185
sausage and Mediterranean
    vegetable sheet pan bake 154
SCOBY 180
sea bass with seaweed salsa
    verde 135
seafood
    Brazilian-style crab 110
    crab spaghetti with seaweed
        101
    Michael's mussels 98
    seafood with seaweed risotto
        139
    shrimp with pasta and seaweed
        138
    squid Provençal 142
    terra mare salad 88
    Thai shrimp with coconut milk
        and seaweed 141
seaweed
    baked salmon with seaweed
        pesto 132
    crab spaghetti with seaweed
        101

dry coconut sambal 120
green gazpacho with seaweed
    63
lemon-cilantro hummus
    with seaweed 74
nutrition 17, 88
quick seaweed miso soup 61
salsa verde with seaweed 117
sea bass with seaweed salsa
    verde 135
seafood with seaweed risotto
    139
shrimp with pasta and seaweed
    138
sour cream and seaweed
    muffins 83
Thai-flavored seaweed
    crackers 79
Thai shrimp with coconut milk
    and seaweed 141
tuna and vegetable stir-fry with
    seaweed 109
turmeric spiced omelet with
    seaweed 38
seeds
    bircher muesli with kefir 45
    creamy pineapple smoothie 51
    flaxseed crackers 78
    healthy homemade granola 34
    mug bread 194
    seeded soda bread 196
    Thai-flavored seaweed
        crackers 79
shepherd's pie, Quorn and
    parsnip 148
shrimp
    nutrition 140
    shrimp with pasta and seaweed
        138
    Thai shrimp with coconut milk
        and seaweed 141
slaw, toasted, with halloumi and
    lemony buttermilk dressing 89
sleep quality 20
smoked mackerel and kale
    kedgeree 47
smoked mackerel pâté 75
smoked salmon
    avocado and 46
    ceviche 84
    scrambled eggs with 37
    spread 77
smoothies
    clever gut green 48
    creamy pineapple 51
    Dr. Tim's healthy gut 50
snacks 18, 201
soda bread, seeded 196
soups
    green gazpacho with seaweed
        63
    gut-soothing vegetable bouillon
        60
    pink celeriac and beet soup 64

soups (*cont.*)
  quick seaweed miso soup 61
  satiety and 19
  spicy lentil and tomato soup 62
sour cream and seaweed muffins
  83
sourdough bread, no-knead 198–9
spinach
  clever gut green smoothie 48
  creamy nutmeg spinach 160
  Dr. Tim's healthy gut smoothie
    50
  Quorn and parsnip shepherd's
    pie 148
  shrimp with pasta and seaweed
    138
  spinach and ricotta blinis 80
  spinach dal 112
  toasted slaw with halloumi and
    lemony buttermilk dressing
    89
  warm lentil salad 87
squid
  Provençal 142
  terra mare salad 88
starch, resistant 40, 41, 176
steak with guacamole and
  blistered tomatoes 153
stir-fries
  green banana and pepper
    stir-fry 163
  marinated tofu stir-fry with
    noodles 144
  tuna and vegetable stir-fry with
    seaweed 109
strawberries
  Dr. Tim's healthy gut smoothie
    50
  strawberry chia jam 208
stress 22
sugars 10, 12
sweet potatoes
  purple sweet potato and
    blackberry pie 210
  sweet potato, kale, and cod
    fishcakes 136
sweeteners, artificial 11

temptation 20
terra mare salad 88
Thai-flavored seaweed crackers
  79
Thai shrimp with coconut milk
  and seaweed 138
thiamine 106
tofu
  Chinese noodle jar 70
  kale and tofu scramble 93
  marinated tofu stir-fry with
    noodles 144

tomatoes 24
  Brazilian-style crab 110
  crab spaghetti with seaweed
    101
  eggplant parmigiana 96
  full English breakfast with
    green bananas 41
  green gazpacho with seaweed
    63
  lentil and tomato soup 62
  Quorn and parsnip shepherd's
    pie 148
  sausage and Mediterranean
    sheet pan bake 154
  slow-roasted tomatoes 172
  squid Provençal 142
  steak with guacamole and
    blistered tomatoes 153
  turkey and mushroom
    bolognese 131
  vegetable and paneer curry
    145
  vegetable-rich tomato sauce
    168
  warm lentil salad 87
tuna and vegetable stir-fry with
  seaweed 109
turkey and mushroom bolognese
  131
turmeric
  dry coconut sambal 120
  nutrition 17
  onion and eggplant bhajis 162
  tea 21
  turmeric buttermik dressing
    119
  turmeric coronation chicken
    111
  turmeric spiced omelet with
    seaweed 38

variety 8
vegetables *see also specific*
vegetables
  Chinese noodle jar 70
  cruciferous 94
  fermented pickled vegetables
    187
  Japanese-style quick-pickled
    vegetables 167
  nightshade family 24
  phyto salad 66–7
  quick garlic-fried greens 161
  roasted Mediterranean
    vegetables, pearl barley, and
    eggs 105
  sausage and Mediterranean
    sheet pan bake 154
  variety 11, 14, 17
  vegetable and paneer curry 145

vegetable bouillon 60
vegetable-rich tomato sauce
  168
Veira's cilantro chicken with
  yogurt and fennel 128

walnuts
  chocolate and walnut bites
    202
  chocolate eggplant cake 202
  exotic carrot cake 205
  mug bread 194
water intake 19
watercress
  blood orange salad with toasted
    coriander 55
  green gazpacho with seaweed
    63
  smoked salmon ceviche 84
weight control 11, 20
willpower 20

xanthan gum 13

yogurt 32
  beet and yogurt dip 72
  with chia jam and toasted
    pistachios 35
  clever gut green smoothie 48
  Dr. Tim's healthy gut smoothie
    50
  with granola and diced pear 32
  lemon-cilantro hummus with
    seaweed 74
  nutrition 17
  smoked mackerel pâté 75
  Veira's cilantro chicken with
    yogurt and fennel 128
yuzu juice, smoked salmon
  ceviche 84

zucchini
  baked salmon with seaweed
    pesto 132
  crab spaghetti with seaweed
    101
  onion and zucchini bhajis 162
  pan-fried zucchini spaghetti
    177
  pasta with pistachio pesto 99
  pickled with mustard seeds 188
  roasted Mediterranean
    vegetables, pearl barley, and
    eggs 105
  sausage and Mediterranean
    sheet pan bake 154
  turkey and mushroom
    bolognese 131
  warm red rice salad with
    zucchini 90